Dysphagia in
Movement Disorders

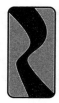

Clinical Dysphagia Series

John C. Rosenbek and Harrison N. Jones
Series Editors

Dysphagia Following Stroke by Stephanie K. Daniels and Maggie-Lee Huckabee
Dysphagia in Movement Disorders by John C. Rosenbek and Harrison N. Jones

Dysphagia in Movement Disorders

A Volume in the Clinical Dysphagia Series

John C. Rosenbek
Harrison N. Jones

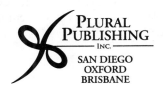

PLURAL
PUBLISHING
INC.

SAN DIEGO
OXFORD
BRISBANE

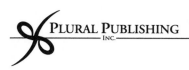

5521 Ruffin Road
San Diego, CA 92123

e-mail: info@pluralpublishing.com
Web site: http://www.pluralpublishing.com

49 Bath Street
Abingdon, Oxfordshire OX14 1EA
United Kingdom

Library of Congress Cataloging-in-Publication Data:

Rosenbek, John C., 1940–
    Dysphagia in movement disorders / John C. Rosenbek & Harrison N. Jones.
      p. ; cm. — (Clinical dysphagia series)
    Includes bibliographical references and index.
    ISBN-13: 978-1-59756-228-7 (alk. paper)
    ISBN-10: 1-59756-228-9 (alk. paper)
    1. Deglutition disorders. 2. Movement disorders –Complications. I. Jones, Harrison N
II. Title. III. Series.
    [DNLM: 1. Deglutition Disorders—diagnosis. 2. Deglutition Disorders—therapy.
3. Deglutition—physiology. 4. Movement Disorders—complications. 5. Movement
Disorders—therapy. WI 250 R813d 2008]
    RC815.2.R67 2008
    616.3'23—dc22
                                                                2008027130

Contents

Foreword

Movement disorders in their various clinical manifestations represent some of the most complex, poorly understood, and clinically challenging conditions encountered by speech-language pathologists. Unfortunately, most descriptions of movement disorders focus primarily on manifestations of those conditions on limb function with little attention given to descriptions of concomitant communicative impairments and swallowing disorders. Consequently it is often left to clinicians to try to predict the effects of movement disorders on functioning of craniofacial structures by extrapolation of clinical findings and descriptions of the effects of these conditions on limb physiology. Adding to the complexity is the fact that movement disorders often have different effects on limb versus craniofacial structures, such as those involved in the oropharyngeal phase of swallowing. In spite of the obvious importance of swallowing impairments to the care and management of persons with movement disorders, their presence is often overlooked or at best only noted in descriptions of various movement disorders without any information provided as to the nature of the swallowing impairment, the assessment procedures to be applied, possible treatment strategies, and overall implications for patient care. As a direct outcome of this neglect, until now there has been little published information to guide clinicians as to the presence and nature of swallowing disorders associated with movement disorders, let alone recommendations for their assessment and treatment.

Despite the lack of published research, in writing the present book, Rosenbek and Jones have successfully compiled a unique volume that will provide clinicians with an unprecedented guide to the diagnosis, assessment, and management of swallowing impairments associated with a wide variety of movement disorders. The present volume is clearly written with clinicians in mind and will serve as a valuable handbook and clinical guide for all clinicians who encounter persons with movement disorders and associated swallowing impairment as part of their clinical practice. Specifically, the book provides comprehensive coverage of all aspects of swallowing associated with movement disorders ranging from basic definitions through clinical and instrumental assessment procedures, principles of compensatory treatments and rehabilitation techniques, to descriptions of swallowing impairments associated with specific movement disorders such as Parkinson's disease, chorea, tremor, ataxic syndromes, and dystonia, to name but a few. Importantly, the recommended evaluations and treatment approaches are set out in an easy to follow, step-by-step fashion to facilitate application of the materials in a real-world clinical setting. Wherever necessary, an overview of the medical and clinical manifestations of each movement disorder is provided and major features outlined in terms of potential influence on swallowing function.

I have no doubt that this unique, well-written, and easy to read book will become not only critical reading but also a long-term essential resource for any speech-language pathologist involved in the care and management of persons with movement disorders.

Professor Bruce Murdoch
School of Health and
  Rehabilitation Sciences
The University of Queensland,
  Australia

Preface

Charles Frazier, the author of *Thirteen Moons*, has his main character, Will Cooper, say: "I cannot decide whether it is an illness or a sin, the need to write things down." We cannot decide either. Perhaps it is both.

If it is illness, then that illness is madness. No other word describes acceptance of a book contract when one of us was chair of a department approaching the worst budget crises in a state's recent history and when the other was trying to complete a doctorate in rehabilitation science. No other word describes what it takes to delay or ignore other pressing intellectual obligations and the simple activities of daily living like being on time, being prepared, being generous. No other word describes acting as if an hour at the end of long days and a few hours on the weekend were what love requires. What better descriptor for two who would promise to write a book on movement disorders and swallowing when even the proper classification of the movement disorders is in flux and when data on swallowing characteristics in most disorders are sparse and treatment data nearly nonexistent?

To make this clinical book, we drew on the data we could find, on what we hope are general principles of evaluation and treatment, and—most extensively—on our years of clinical experience: 38 for one and 10 for the other. As hard as we tried, we did not completely avoid sin during the writing. We know readers will discover sins of omission—literature not cited, authors and clinicians inadequately acknowledged, disorders not mentioned. Sins of commission are probably even more abundant, misinterpretations, bad guesses, premature conclusions, and recommendations inadequately supported by data and experience.

We set out to write a clinical book. We tried to format the content so busy clinicians could find useful information quickly. We tried to restrict that content to the most clinically relevant. We tried to cite sufficient literature so that interested readers can go farther into nearly every topic if their practices require it. As clinicians ourselves, we constantly asked ourselves if the words we were writing had a chance of easing the clinical burden for working clinicians in busy, diverse practices.

Now it is done. We can already feel our sanity returning. As for our sins— they are now public. We apologize for them in advance.

John C. Rosenbek
Harrison N. Jones

ix

JCR: *For the three women who make everything possible—*
Debra, Wendy, and Vaughn

HNJ: *For Carlee and Nate, "Big" Mike and Linda*

1 Purpose and Scope

This is a clinical book about swallowing. Swallowing is the complex activity of suspending respiration while moving saliva, food, drink, or any other substance from the mouth through the pharynx and esophagus into the stomach. Traditionally, the nonrespiratory portion of this complex process is divided into oropharyngeal and esophageal stages. An appalling number of congenital and acquired conditions can disrupt the process, resulting in what are commonly referred to as either *oropharyngeal* or *esophageal* dysphagias. This book is dedicated to *oropharyngeal dysphagia in adults resulting from movement disorders*.

This book is intended for the clinician and for clinical use. It is written to support understanding, evaluation, and behavioral treatment of the swallowing problems resulting from the full range of movement disorders, such as Parkinson's disease (PD), multiple system atrophy (MSA), Huntington's disease (HD), and dystonia. Our wish is that if a patient with even a rare movement disorder appears in the clinic, this book will offer some guidance.

Separate chapters are devoted to specific disorders such as PD or to classes of movement disorder such as ataxia and dystonia. In these general chapters such as the entry on dystonia, individual conditions such as Meige syndrome will appear alongside other conditions. This organization was chosen because so little is known about swallowing in most of the disorders characterized by movement abnormality. PD is an obvious exception; hence, this condition has its own chapter. Even the general chapters differ in length, depending on what is known. These chapters have the same organization, including definitions, disorders, epidemiology, general and swallowing signs and symptoms, and special evaluative and treatment considerations. The evaluation and management options are based on the evidence, when it exists, our own clinical experiences, and the realities of the modern health care environment.

The book begins with short chapters on definitions; anatomy and physiology of the normal swallow; the history and chart review; and the clinical, videofluoroscopic, and videoendoscopic swallowing examinations. These chapters are followed by entries outlining general and specific principles governing behavioral management and discussions of behavioral treatments divided, with some trepidation, into rehabilitative and compensatory approaches. The disorder chapters comprise the book's final section. The book ends with appendices of particularly useful information.

This book is meant for the practitioner. Where clinical arguments about what to expect or do exist, we take a stand. Where nothing is known for sure, we take a chance. These are the same stands and chances we take in our own clinical practices.

2 Definitions and Classifications

Normal swallowing and dysphagia are defined in this chapter. The stages of swallowing, a traditional conceit that fits only uncomfortably with the act of moving food and drink from the mouth to the stomach, are also described briefly. In some instances a movement disorder may disproportionately affect one stage or another; therefore, we have preserved the idea of stages. Clinicians are asked to recognize, however, that the majority of swallowing problems affect more than one stage and that these divisions are somewhat arbitrary (Martin-Harris, Michel, & Castell, 2005). The second section of this chapter is devoted to a discussion of definition and classification in movement disorders. The problems of classification of these disorders have never been solved to everyone's satisfaction. Certainly, our solution will not be universally applauded. It works for us clinically so we have used it here.

NORMAL SWALLOWING

Normal swallowing is the complex cognitive, sensorimotor act of moving any bolus from the mouth to the stomach. Normal swallows are *safe*, *efficient*, and *satisfying*.

Stages of Swallowing

Swallowing, traditionally, is divided into four stages: oral preparatory, oral, pharyngeal, and esophageal. The *oral preparatory stage* is highly volitional and characterized by chewing and mixing the bolus with saliva. The *oral stage* is characterized by the final formation of the bolus into a convenient shape and posterior movement of that bolus through the faucial pillars and into the pharynx to trigger the pharyngeal stage of swallowing. For our purposes, we generally combine the oral preparatory stage and the oral stage and have done so throughout this book. In the *pharyngeal stage*, the bolus is moved through the pharynx and rostral esophagus. This striated muscle section of the esophagus is called the upper esophageal sphincter (UES). The *esophageal stage* involves movement of the bolus through the esophagus into the stomach. It is useful to think of these stages as overlapping and interacting in what can be seen as a complex, sequential response. It is also common to view the stages as existing along a continuum of automaticity, with the esophageal stage being most automatic and the oral preparatory stage the least.

DYSPHAGIA

Dysphagia is defined as *disordered movement of the bolus from mouth to stomach due to abnormalities in the structures critical to swallowing or in their movements*. Dysphagia involving any one or combination of the stages can make swallowing unsafe and put a patient at risk for malnutrition, dehydration, fatal choking episodes, and pulmonary consequences of aspiration. It can make the swallow inefficient and require that the patient take hours to eat. It can make eating unpleasant because the patient fears choking or grows weary of dietary restrictions.

Normal Movement

Normal movement depends minimally on *posture, strength, timing, tone, steadiness*, and *praxis* or *skill*.

Movement Disorders

Classic neurology identifies a set of movement disorders, although all textbooks and practitioners do not agree on all the appropriate members of this set. Fernandez, Rodriguez, Skidmore, and Okun (2007) begin by categorizing all movement abnormalities as either hyperkinetic, characterized by an excess of movement, or hypokinetic, characterized by a "paucity" of movement. For these authors, the two main *hypokinetic* abnormalities are what they call *parkinsonism* and *rigidity*, whereas the *hyperkinetic* abnormalities are *chorea, dystonia, myoclonus, tic,* and *tremor*. Restless leg syndrome is also included as a major component of

the hyperkinetic conditions, but no further mention of it will occur in this book on swallowing. Experienced clinicians recognize that other often-identified movement abnormalities such as athetosis and ballismus are absent from the list. Fernandez and colleagues (2007) include these two with chorea and opine that these three abnormalities may actually exist on a continuum.

It is unclear how most of these conditions affect swallowing and if their effects are unique. Clinical experience suggests that some of these abnormalities (e.g., tic) have less frequent and disastrous effects on swallowing than do others (such as Parkinson's disease [PD]). For all, the severity of the abnormality may determine the swallowing effect, as may the coexistence of other abnormalities such as weakness.

Modern clinical neurology usually begins with an emphasis on the disease state (i.e., disorder) such as PD or multiple system atrophy (MSA) rather than movement abnormalities per se. The movement abnormalities are used primarily in support of the movement disorder diagnosis. Logic would seem to dictate individual chapters on each of the movement disorders. Unfortunately, that approach was unworkable. More than one hundred movement disorders have been identified. Some, such as PD, are frequent and the resulting dysphagia has been widely studied. Others, such as MSA, are more rarely encountered and dysphagia is less well studied. The result would have been an inordinate number of chapters of wildly varying lengths and specificity.

Equally unworkable would have been chapters devoted to each of the movement abnormalities. The rarity of some is but one complication. In addition, some such as tic often have no influence on swallowing. More critical is that some conditions that are traditionally regarded as movement disorders (such as PD) may present with most of the abnormal movements listed. Likewise, some abnormalities such as tremor may be present in a majority of the commonly recognized disease states.

Therefore, the chapter headings in this volume are a mixture of diseases (e.g., PD, Wilson's disease [WD]) and of movement abnormalities (chorea, dystonia, dyskinesia). Given this format, the Index will often serve as a better guide to the content than will the Table of Contents.

As is obvious from the foregoing, movement disorders present as many challenges for the writer as for the clinician. We try to counter that difficulty a bit by being as specific about how to identify and manage the swallowing disorders of those with movement disorders as our experience and the data allow.

3 Swallowing Anatomy and Physiology

Understanding swallowing anatomy and physiology makes for better clinical practice. Topics of this chapter are (a) swallowing structures, (b) muscle systems, (c) neural system control of normal swallowing, and (d) general sequence of activities during the normal swallow. Knowing this information guides the diagnostician who must make sense of an abnormal swallow and the rehabilitationist who must select an appropriate treatment.

The major structures of swallowing, some of which are made solely of muscle, are shown in Figure 3–1.

A brief summary of the contributions of these structures to swallowing are provided in Table 3–1.

The clinician can expect these structures to be intact in patients with

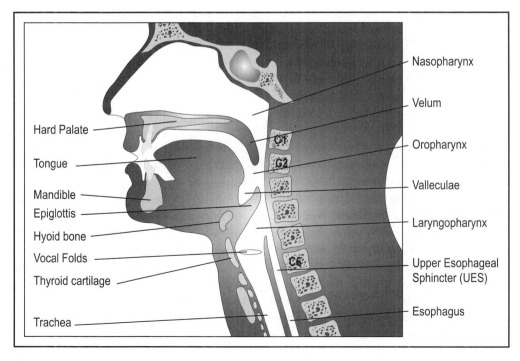

Figure 3–1. Critical structures involved in swallowing.

Hard Palate
Tongue
Mandible
Epiglottis
Hyoid bone
Vocal Folds
Thyroid cartilage
Trachea

Nasopharynx
Velum
Oropharynx
Valleculae
Laryngopharynx
Upper Esophageal Sphincter (UES)
Esophagus

C1
C2
C6

Table 3–1. Major structures and their contributions to swallowing

Mandible	Stabilizes all swallowing structures and opens mouth
Maxilla	Forms roof of mouth
Lips	Anterior seal
Teeth	Bolus preparation
Cheeks	Support bolus preparation and movement
Soft palate	Separates mouth and nose when elevated during swallow
Pharynx	Forms swallowing tube between mouth and upper esophageal sphincter Muscles contract to help propel the bolus
Hyoid bone	Provides critical attachments for supra- and infrahyoid muscles
Larynx	Cartilaginous infrastructure for intrinsic and extrinsic laryngeal musculature
Spine	Posterior bony support for swallowing musculature
Upper esophageal sphincter (UES)	Striated muscle valve at top of esophagus
Esophagus	Route from pharynx to stomach
Lower esophageal sphincter (LES)	Valve at distal end of esophagus
Lungs and trachea	Major components of respiratory mechanism

movement disorders unless a particular patient has a coexisting disease such as head/neck cancer. Nonetheless, each (with the possible exception of the esophagus, lower esophageal sphincter [LES], and respiratory structures; see Chapters 4–7 on evaluation for more details) should be examined by the dysphagia clinician every time a patient with a movement disorder is referred for a swallowing evaluation. Patients may also present with two conditions, as when a person with cerebellar degeneration also

has large osteophytes obstructing the upper esophageal sphincter (UES). Additionally, the neurologic diagnoses can be wrong or impossible to confirm with confidence.

What is most frequent in movement disorders, of course, is that the movements of these structures rather than the structures themselves will be disrupted. Identifying these movement abnormalities and their contributions to abnormal swallowing is a major obligation if treatments are to succeed.

SWALLOWING MUSCULATURE

The major muscles groups and their principal swallowing functions are included in Table 3–2. Assignment of function is simplified but sufficient to support most clinical problem solving. For more details, consult Corbin-Lewis, Liss, & Sciortino (2005).

The actions of these muscle groups are controlled by the central and peripheral nervous systems. The esophagus is composed primarily of smooth muscles; the oropharynx and respiratory muscles are striated; therefore, neural control of them is somewhat different.

NERVOUS SYSTEM CONTROL

Nervous system control of swallowing movements involves selected sensory and motor branches of specific cranial and spinal nerves (for respiration) and central networks extending from brainstem to cortex. Understanding how swallowing is controlled is especially important for the clinician who sees patients with movement disorders.

Major Peripheral Nerves

The major cranial and spinal nerves important to swallowing are outlined in

Table 3–2. Muscle groups important in swallowing and the contributions their activity make to normal swallowing

Facial	Provide anterior and lateral muscular boundaries of the oral cavity and move jaw
Lingual	Control tongue shape and contribute to movement of the tongue during bolus formation and movement
Palatal	Elevate and lower the soft palate
Pharyngeal	Contribute to bolus flow through the pharynx and UES
Laryngeal	Elevate and close the larynx
Submental	Aid elevation and forward movement of the hyolaryngeal complex
Subhyoid	Contribute to movement of the hyolaryngeal complex
Esophageal	Move bolus into stomach
LES	Control bolus movement into and out of the stomach
Inspiratory muscles	Support sufficient inhalation
Expiratory muscles	Move air and support cough

Table 3–3. These nerves constitute what is often called the *final common pathway*. Their disruption can cause serious swallowing problems because, as the final common pathway, all higher cortical and subcortical effects are channeled through them. Figure 3–2 illustrates the 12 cranial nerves.

Central Pattern Generators

A major contribution to swallowing control resides with bilateral brainstem mechanisms called *central pattern generators* (CPGs; Miller, 1999). CPGs are modifiable by bilateral nervous system components above the brainstem. Nonetheless, they make critical contributions to normal swallowing. The CPGs, one on each side of the medulla, are divided into interacting sensory and motor components.

1. The sensory component or *dorsal sensory division* comprises nucleus solitarius and the surrounding reticular activating system bilaterally. Sensory information, including touch, pressure, and temperature, from the oral cavity and pharynx converge on this nucleus and are organized to influence the sequential motor movements of both respiration and oropharyngeal swallowing.

2. The motor component or *ventral motor division* comprises nucleus ambiguous and surrounding reticular activating system bilaterally. This division is the origin of the patterned nervous impulses that activate the swallowing (and to a degree the respiratory) muscles to perform a coordinated swallow.

Cortical and Subcortical Contributions

Although the brainstem CPGs are capable of controlling swallowing, most human

Nerve	Structure Innervated
Table 3–3. Major cranial and spinal nerves and their contributions to swallowing	
Cranial nerve (CN) V (trigeminal)	Muscles for chewing and sensation from the palate, tongue, and inner cheeks
Cranial nerve VII (facial)	Muscles of face and lips and taste from anterior tongue
Cranial nerve IX (glossopharyngeal)	Sensation from posterior tongue, faucial pillars, and pharynx
Cranial nerve X (vagus)	Muscles of larynx, pharynx, velopharynx
Cranial nerve XII (hypoglossal)	Intrinsic and extrinsic muscles of tongue
Twenty-two spinal nerves are involved in respiration, including 8 cervical nerves, 12 thoracic nerves, and 2 lumbar nerves. Four cranial nerves also make contributions (CNs IX, X, XI, and XII).	The *phrenic nerve*, which comprises branches of C3–C5, innervates the diaphragm. Lower spinal nerves are generally responsible for motor innervation to successively lower regions of the chest wall. Sensory innervation of the chest wall is similarly organized (Hixon & Hoit, 2005).

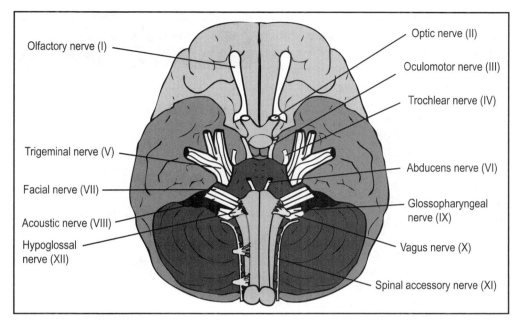

Figure 3–2. The 12 cranial nerves.

swallows receive tuning, modulating, or modifying influences from centers above the brainstem. Mosier and Bereznaya (2001) have presented data suggesting that there are five distinct "clusters" involved in cortical (and subcortical) control for swallowing, which include the following.

1. Primary motor cortex, primary sensory cortex, supplementary motor cortex, and cingulate gyrus
2. Inferior frontal gyrus, secondary sensory cortex, corpus callosum, basal ganglia, and thalamus
3. Premotor cortex and posterior parietal cortex
4. Cerebellum
5. Insula

Knowing this information prepares the clinician for the appearance of dysphagia from involvement nearly any-

where along the neural axis from the myoneural junction, where muscle and nerve interface, through the brainstem and subcortical and cortical structures. As will be seen in subsequent chapters, all these regions, with the possible exception of the myoneural junction and final common pathway, may be involved in one or more of the movement disorders.

ORDER OF SWALLOWING EVENTS

Swallowing is a complex process that is altered by multiple conditions, including bolus size and whether a person is swallowing a single sip or completing serial swallows. It is not disrupted in the same way or to the same degree in all illnesses or even by the same illness in two different people. Therefore, evaluation and treatment depend on identifying individual patterns of abnormality. One guide to that identification is the approximate order of events in a normal swallow. Deviations from that pattern may or may not create bolus flow abnormalities. These events may overlap and occur in different orders for different people and for the same person under different conditions. Recall as well that this order does not matter unless bolus flow abnormalities result that influence the safety, adequacy, or enjoyment of eating.

Martin-Harris and colleagues (2003, 2005) have systematically explored the temporal coordination of swallowing events with breathing. The approximate order of the normal occurrence of these events is shown in Table 3-4. Note the cessation of breathing until near the end of the swallow. Martin-Harris and colleagues use the terminology *pharyngoesophageal segment* (PES) for what we refer to as the UES. This timeline has many clinical implications. One of these implications is that there is a general pattern that is encountered (with some opportunity for variability) in normal swallowing. Additionally, this timeline emphasizes the critical role of respiration in swallowing and suggests that respiratory abnormalities can themselves lead to dysphagia.

The successful clinician can carry knowledge of structures, muscles, neural

Table 3–4. Events in a normal swallow are initiated in approximately this order
Apnea onset
Oral bolus transport
Hyoid excursion
Laryngeal closure
Maximum laryngeal closure
PES opening
Maximum hyoid excursion
Laryngeal opening
Swallowing inspiration
Apnea onset
Last PES opening
Hyoid return

Note. PES = pharyngoesophageal segment

From "Temporal Coordination of Pharyngeal and Laryngeal Dynamics with Breathing during Swallowing: Single Liquid Swallows," by B. Martin-Harris et al., 2003, *Journal of Applied Physiology, 94,* pp. 1735–1743, and "Physiologic Model of Oropharyngeal Swallowing Revisited," by B. Martin-Harris, Y. Michal, and D. O. Castell, 2005, *Otolaryngology– Head and Neck Surgery, 133,* pp. 234–240. Copyright 2003 and 2005.

control, and sequencing of swallowing events into every evaluation and treatment planning session. The results will be increasingly insightful evaluation and explanation and more focused treatment.

4 Chart Review and History

Some very experienced clinicians avoid any chart review except to reassure themselves that the patient is appropriate for some level of evaluation and to find out about any special precautions for clinician and patient safety. They do so to avoid being biased during their own examination. In general, we do not support this approach, preferring instead a thorough chart review that may actually alert us to multiple diagnostic and therapeutic possibilities. Doing so, of course, requires vigilance lest one be seduced into discovering only what one expects. What is one looking for in such a review?

TYPES OF INFORMATION

General Information

General information is important to record keeping and insurance claims and can even help with planning management. A minimum data set would include:

1. Patient name
2. Insurance information including eligibility for services
3. Age
4. Gender
5. Handedness
6. Education

7. Socioeconomic status
8. Present and/or past employment
9. Present activities and responsibilities
10. Place of residence and living situation

Clinical/Medical Information

The chart can be a rich source of information in support of both diagnostic and therapeutic procedures. This information is of several overlapping types:

1. Information to aid diagnosis
2. Information to aid prognosis
3. Information to aid treatment planning
4. Information to aid selection of best measure of treatment outcome
5. Information to aid decisions about referral

SOURCES OF INFORMATION

Chart Review

Obviously, information from the chart review can serve more than one of these purposes. Consequently, a list of the most essential information from the medical record is featured below. The list begins with *general medical history* and then moves to *specific swallowing related*

13

history. More disorder-specific questions are included in the chapters devoted to each of the movement disorder diagnoses. For all patients, we recommend searching the chart for the following.

General Medical History

Presumed Medical Diagnosis and Diagnostician. The various movement disorders have different signs, symptoms, and prognoses. Additionally, these conditions likely require different medical/surgical and behavioral treatments. For example, Parkinson's disease (PD) and multiple system atrophy (MSA) have different signs, and MSA is less responsive to medical management and behavioral treatments. Additionally, some diagnosticians are more likely to be correct than others. Most would agree that movement disorders are most likely to be properly diagnosed by a fellowship-trained movement disorders neurologist. In other words, a clinician's confidence in the medical diagnosis may vary depending on the diagnostician.

Time of Onset. Some conditions, such as Wilson's disease (WD), occur more frequently in younger than older persons, a fact which can aid diagnosis. In all movement disorders, the onset of symptoms may occur weeks, months, or years prior to diagnosis, and an early diagnosis can be wrong. Tremor due to PD, for example, can be misdiagnosed as essential tremor. Unfortunately, the wrong therapy can also be delivered prior to establishing a correct diagnosis. Finally, early behavioral treatment may be more beneficial than later intervention, although this is a notion in search of data.

Signs at Onset. Signs at onset can aid prognosis and diagnosis. It may be that right-sided signs such as right arm tremor are associated with the more rapid onset of speech and swallowing symptoms, although this remains an experimental question.

Course of Signs. Disease courses are of three main types: stable, deteriorating, and improving. Deterioration is the usual course of movement disorders, though the rate of decline varies considerably across diseases and even within a disease. Generally, a rapidly progressive disease is less amenable to treatment than is one with a more indolent course. Treatment, however, should never be denied simply on the basis of rapidity of decline. Even if rehabilitation is impossible, compensations can be tried. If treatment is offered, frequent changes in goals and procedures may be necessary, especially in rapidly worsening disease. Special vigilance is important in persons with rapid decline, especially for those with dysphagia, as life-threatening consequences can occur quickly.

Variability of Signs. Identifying, when possible, the positive and negative influences on signs can be clinically useful because some of the negative influences may be modifiable and the positive ones can be reinforced. Possible influences include time of day, fatigue, activity, anxiety, medications and medication schedule, and sensory tricks (see dystonia chapter for more details). Clinicians can obtain this information by asking, "What makes your problems (and it is usually best to list specific ones such as swallowing) better? What makes them worse?" If a patient is unsure, then providing examples such as time of day, medications, and fatigue can be helpful. Because medications can be the most powerful influence on behavior, having a list of the medications and their schedule, including the date of initiation, can be important, as can be the date(s) of any surgical interventions.

Planned, Completed, or Ongoing Medical or Surgical Management. Infrequently, a clinician will see an individual with a movement disorder prior to the initiation of any other treatment. Evaluation is still appropriate and may even contribute to medical diagnosis. Behavioral treatment for such a patient, however, is seldom appropriate unless no medical or surgical treatments are planned. In general, it is preferable to withhold behavioral treatments until after medical and surgical effects can be evaluated. A possible exception to this is the simultaneous initiation of medical/surgical and behavioral treatments. With the growing interest in the potential *neuroprotective* effects of exercise, such early, simultaneous treatments may become more frequent. Neuroprotective as used here means that an exercise may slow a disease's progress.

Success of Medical or Surgical Treatment. Many movement disorders are responsive to medications and/or surgery; some are not. The best example of a good responder is PD, which often responds positively for years to medications and subsequently to deep brain stimulation (DBS). Frequently, this response will be confined to functions supported by the corticospinal system such as limb movements. Corticobulbar functions such as speech and swallowing are often unaffected or in some instances made worse, an observation to which we will return. Treating the unresponsive patient with behavioral methods is challenging because the prognosis is usually only fair at best. Clinicians should not avoid such patients,

however, as compensations can sometimes make a difference. The ideal situation is to pair successful medical and/or surgical approaches with behavioral ones.

Side Effects of Medical/Surgical and Behavioral Management. Over time, both medical and surgical treatments can lose their effectiveness. For example, in patients with PD, levodopa therapy usually becomes less beneficial over time and may be associated with "on-off" effects and dyskinesia. Another example is decline of bulbar function following DBS surgery in some patients. These unfortunate side effects complicate the lives of those with movement disorders and present special challenges for clinicians. As such, they influence treatment planning and prognosis.

Other Medical Problems. Seldom does an adult patient have only one condition. Therefore, assembling a so-called problem list as a basis for understanding the patient's overall medical condition and for determining why the patient has dysphagia is important. Space does not permit summarizing all the conditions capable of causing or contributing to dysphagia. The wise diagnostician will be careful to rule out such conditions as esophageal dysmotility (when trying to explain an oropharyngeal dysphagia), xerostomia from medications, and so on. All reasons must be addressed by appropriate professionals. If they cannot be, then prognosis dims.

Swallowing History

It is increasingly likely that some swallowing history will be included in the chart. What follows are data especially important to treatment planning.

Onset and Course of Swallowing Problems. Onset and course will give the clinician insight into the rapidity of decline. In general, indolent courses provide greater opportunity for rehabilitation, although this is not absolute. Relatively recent onset may leave a person wondering if the swallowing problem is the result of the movement diagnosis or of some other condition. Recent onset and steep decline generally suggest a poorer prognosis.

Weight Loss. Weight loss may signal the severity of the dysphagia if evaluation confirms swallowing function as a primary influence on weight. Weight loss from malnutrition may contribute to the severity of the dysphagia because of malnutrition's negative impact on muscle function. Weight loss, from whatever cause, signals the need for a dietician to join the treatment team. Malnutrition darkens prognosis for improvement in all functions, and a feeding tube may be suggested to help normalize nutrition and hydration parameters prior to initiation of behavioral treatment.

Pneumonia. A history of pneumonia, especially in a dysphagic person with aspiration, suggests more pneumonias are likely unless the dysphagia is addressed. It is important to note that, even in those with dysphagia, not all pneumonias result from the aspiration of food and drink. A person with a history of pneumonia, from whatever cause, needs the most aggressive possible team treatment.

Other Medical and Health Consequences. A variety of other sequelae can flow from or be associated with dysphagia. Of special interest are loss of interest in eating, changes in diet and in eating behavior (e.g., no longer going out to eat or avoiding eating with others), fear of eating, depression, weight loss, and having required the Heimlich maneuver. The clinical challenge is in discovering which of these conditions result from the dysphagia and which have other etiologies. Anorexia, medication effects, and depression may be as important as dysphagia in explaining why a person is not eating, for example. Indeed, the only member of this list that most assuredly results from dysphagia is having required a Heimlich maneuver.

Relation of Medical/Surgical Treatments to Swallowing. The need is to establish the relationship, if any, of medical or surgical interventions to swallowing difficulty. If swallowing is worse as a result, then the likelihood of improving it is diminished. Treatment is still indicated but expectations need to be muted. Conversely, if medical or surgical treatment improves swallowing, then behavioral treatment may be unnecessary. If it is indicated, the prognosis for further improvement may be enhanced. The history and the appropriate scheduling of evaluation (before and after surgery, at various times in the medication cycle) are the best guides to the relationship of medical and surgical treatments to swallowing competence.

History

Recall that the above discussion has to do with the chart review. Some of the previously described information may not be in the chart, the chart may be unavailable or incomplete, or some information may be wrong. However, even if all the information is present, the patient and caregiver should be queried for confirmation and clarification. Of special interest, and often not available in the medical record, are the following.

Time and Conditions under which Swallowing Symptoms Appeared

The longer the duration of dysphagia, the less reliable the history and the greater is the treatment challenge.

Medical Conditions at Onset Can Also Help to Confirm Etiology

It warrants remembering that patients can have two or more diseases or conditions and mistakes can occur from the reflexive assignment of all signs to the disease for which the patient is being referred.

Course of Deficit

Some conditions deteriorate rapidly and some much less so. Prognosis and the need for more or less aggressive intervention can be guided by these different courses.

Difficult Food and Liquid Items

This can be a fairly exhaustive set of questions. This information helps to confirm the severity and functional and health impact of the dysphagia. This may also guide selection of testing materials for those clinicians at liberty to test a portion of the foods patients complain of difficulty with. If patient complains of food sticking, then get identification of level and when it occurs—early, late, or variably during meals and non-eating periods. Food sticking lower in the chest may suggest esophageal involvement. Food sticking at the level of the larynx more likely

implicates the oropharynx, though this complaint may be esophageal in nature as well. Food sticking late during meals also may implicate esophagus rather than oropharynx.

Foods and Liquids Dropped from Diet

This may help establish functional significance and give insight into need for consultation with a dietician. Additionally, we have found that this may be helpful in generating goals for treatment. For example, being able to return to eating a favorite food can be a motivating treatment goal.

Length of Time Needed to Eat

This can be a very useful functional measure of dysphagia's impact on swallowing-related quality of life. This can also be used as a functional swallowing measure if a standardized, safe food choice can be prepared.

Importance of Dysphagia in the Overall Symptom Complex

This is a powerful motivator of treatment, in that treatment is most urgent in those with dysphagia at or near the top of their symptom profile. This may help direct the entire team to the hierarchy of treatments to deliver.

Impact on Quality of Life

This is the best indicator of the consequences of the dysphagia and a strong motivator for participation in treatment. Additionally, this is the best indicator of the actual functional consequences of the disorder regardless of what clinical measures may indicate.

What Makes Swallowing Better or Worse

This provides insight into potential compensatory manipulations such as slower eating, altered posture, or altered diet. Prognosis is better in those cases where improvement is possible.

Influence on Swallowing of any Medical or Surgical Treatments

If these treatments worsen swallowing, then prognosis with behavioral treatment is dimmed. This is also an indication that behavioral treatment may be the last, and best, hope for improvement.

Pneumonia and Date(s) of Occurrence

A history of pneumonia is a predictor of subsequent pneumonias. A history positive for frequent pneumonia indicates the need for aggressive rehabilitation, all other things being equal. This may also suggest extreme conservatism in recommendations.

Choking Episodes per Meal, Day, Week, or Month

The frequency of choking episodes may be one of best indicators of severity. At the very least, this signals the clinician that teaching the Heimlich maneuver to family or other caregivers is important.

Weight Loss

Table 4-1 provides a list of possible reasons for weight loss. Weight loss may also potentially be an indicator of severity. Significant weight loss may generate the need for aggressive rehabilitation, dietary

Table 4–1. Possible reasons for weight loss

Early satiety

Depression

Psychiatric illness

Limited or unappealing food choices

Impaired taste, smell, or ability to bring food to mouth

Poverty, isolation

Anorexia of aging

Poorly fitting or absent dentures

Medications suppressing appetite

Dementia

Alcoholism

Other addictions

Note. From "The Anorexia of Aging in Adults," by N. P. Hays and S. B. Roberts, 2006, *Physiology & Behavior, 88,* pp. 257–266; "Pathophysiology of Anorexia," by J. E. Morley, 2002, *Clinics in Geriatric Medicine, 18,* pp. 661–673; and "Nutritional Evaluation and Laboratory Values in Dysphagia Management," by V. Zachary and R. H. Mills, 2000, in R. H. Mills (Ed.), *Evaluation of Dysphagia in Adult: Expanding the Diagnostic Options* (pp. 179–206), Austin, TX: PRO-ED, Inc.

consultation, and careful evaluation of all factors that influence weight loss.

Heimlich Maneuvers Required

This sounds the alarm about the need for aggressive management and provides the best indication of the health consequences of the dysphagia. Knowing the frequency helps to direct the treatment, including prognosis and treatment planning. Additionally, it should be ensured that the patient and caregivers understand the Heimlich maneuver.

Special Concerns about Drooling

Drooling is a sensitive sign of oropharyngeal dysphagia that directs the clinician to explore all reasons in addition to dysphagia that may explain drooling. Drooling is often very distressing to the patient and family and it is likely to be important to the patient's evaluation of treatment success.

Difficulty with Swallowing Saliva

If reported at night, inquire about a wet pillow upon rising in the morning. Additionally, attempt to determine whether this occurs on the right, left, or both ends of the patient's pillow. This may provide some information about laterality. If difficulty swallowing saliva occurs during the day, it supports an organic etiology, because this almost never occurs in psychogenic conditions. This also strongly suggests that the problem is oropharyngeal unless accompanied by signs of esophageal deficit such as belching, chest pain, and reflux.

Patient and Family Expectations Regarding Evaluation

Patient or family expectations are critical in that they direct the clinician to goals. Treatment is more likely to be beneficial if the patient and family goals are addressed. Clinicians can expect to meet these goals if they are realistic and if a treatment is available that targets them. If goals are unrealistic and the family and patient's expectations cannot be modified, the clinician can expect that treatment will not be seen as successful by patient and family.

Acceptance and Expectations of Treatment for the Swallowing Disorder

Patients must accept treatment or nothing permanent will be accomplished. Expectations such as relief from the feeling of food sticking will aid the clinician's planning of what to measure as a treatment success.

History of Previous Treatment for Dysphagia Including Effects

Previous treatments and their benefit (or lack thereof) may provide prognostic information in that if a patient reports previous significant profit, significant benefit, under usual circumstances, can be expected again. This information on what approaches have been tried and their relative success will also aid in treatment planning. A clinician usually is advised not to retry something that already is perceived as having failed. On the other hand, if successful, then the likelihood that another treatment will also succeed is increased.

Energy Level

Fatigue is a frequent complaint in patients with movement disorders, which may well influence performance and prognosis. SWAL-QOL provides quantification of fatigue (see below and Appendix A).

Amount of Activity

This is measured simply as an estimate of amount of time sitting or lying. The more activity, the better the prognosis. Increased activity may facilitate learning in therapy and can even be a therapeutic goal.

Sleeping Pattern

This is minimally calculated as an estimate of number of hours asleep and number of times awake during the night. This may likely influence prognosis, given that good sleep appears to be related to prognosis for improving with instruction.

A SPECIAL TEST FOR MEASURING DYSPHAGIA— SPECIFIC QUALITY OF LIFE

The SWAL-QOL is a 44-item quality of life scale specific to dysphagia across 10 quality of life domains and an additional section on symptom frequency (McHorney, Bricker, Kramer, et al., 2000; McHorney, Bricker, Robbins, et al., 2000; McHorney, Robbins, Lomax, et al., 2002; McHorney, Martin-Harris, Robbins, & Rosenbek, 2006). The 10 domains are burden, eating duration, eating desire, food selection, communication, fear, mental health, social role, fatigue, and sleep. The symptom scale comprises 14 symptoms including coughing, choking, gagging, and drooling. Each domain is sampled with a minimum of two items on a five-point scale. The higher the score, the better the dysphagia-related quality of life. Symptom frequency is also scored on a five-point scale. The SWAL-QOL scale can be found in Appendix A.

SWAL-QOL was developed using a wide variety of patients, including those with movement disorders. Thus, it can be used with all such patients. It is included in this chapter because it is scored by the patient unless disability makes reading and responding impossible. In this latter case, a family member or other caregiver can complete the form. It is a psychometrically sound measure that allows the patient to quantify the experience of having a swallowing disorder, and it quantifies a portion of the history.

SWAL-QOL takes an average of 20 minutes to complete. To preserve its psychometric properties, it should be mailed to the patient prior to the visit and completed prior to the visit. Obviously, this tool is developed for outpatients. The reason for that limitation was that inpatients may not be able to appreciate the full range of quality of life impacts of their dysphagia because they are in a protected environment. In addition, a person must be taking something by mouth to make the scoring valid. Patients receiving tube feedings are not excluded, so long as they are taking at least some nourishment by mouth.

Results add quantification to the history and can be included in the report. We include all scores in the results section of the report, because we have developed a template for this and all other measures. We then discuss their implication in the discussion (see Chapter 8 for more details regarding the report).

USE OF THE DATA

A chart review and history, including data from SWAL-QOL, provide critical information. The likelihood and effect of dysphagia, its onset, and course are certainly suggested and for the experienced clinician may be confirmed. The data also aid prognosis and treatment planning. Indeed, a reasonably complete picture of the dysphagia and the person with the condition emerge from these data. Treatment cannot be planned or conducted solely on the basis of the chart review and history. However, the urgency and focus of further examination and treatment can be derived.

The issue of treatment planning deserves special discussion. The presence of swallowing abnormality, if it has functional consequences for a person, even in the absence of health consequences such as pneumonia, must be treated. The chart review and history may confirm functional consequences. The treatment approach, however, may depend upon an instrumented examination, usually the videofluoroscopic swallow examination (VFSE).

The other urgency for swallowing treatment is the presence or likelihood of an illness resulting from the dysphagia. That a person has a history of aspiration pneumonia, which is but one example of a health consequence of dysphagia, is usually discoverable from the history. The chart review and history can even provide key pieces of data about the individual patient's likelihood of illness subsequent to aspiration. It is, after all, the documented occurrence or threat of illness that can be most critical in swallowing management, because preventing illness is of paramount clinical importance.

Let us consider the clinical challenge of predicting illness. It is not as simple as merely identifying a history of aspiration. Aspiration is a critical prerequisite to illness, of course, but all individuals who aspirate do not fall ill. Although much more work is to be done to improve prediction, extant data provide a solid beginning. Table 4–2 contains a summary of predictors of illness from aspiration from the work of Langmore and colleagues (1998).

Table 4–2. Variables associated with aspiration pneumonia in 189 elderly veterans in a variety of settings including outpatients, inpatients, and nursing home residents

Variables Associated with Aspiration Pneumonia

Medical/Health Status

Diagnosis of stroke or other neurologic disease, COPD, GI disease, and CHF

Nursing home resident

Currently smoking

Multiple medical diagnoses

Number of medications

Functional Status

Dependent for oral care

Dependent for feeding*

Dysphagia and GE Reflux Status

Dysphagia and aspiration

Aspiration of food

Pharyngeal swallow delay and postswallow pharyngeal residue

Aspiration of secretions

Excess oral secretions

Reduced esophageal motility

Mode of Nutritional Intake

Tube feeding

Oral/Dental Status

Number of decayed teeth

Frequency of brushing teeth

Dependent for oral care

*Most significant predictor of pneumonia.

Note. From "Predictors of Aspiration Pneumonia: How Important Is Dysphagia?" by S. E. Langmore, M. S. Terpenning, A. Schork, Y. Chen, J. T. Murray, et al., 1998, *Dysphagia, 13,* pp. 69–81.

The variables listed in Table 4–2 influence health in several ways:

1. Dysphagia: Dysphagia increases the likelihood of a patient's aspirating.
2. Colonization: The oral cavity is a potential source of infection that can be aspirated into the lungs.
3. Reduced pulmonary clearance: Aspiration is especially threatening if the patient is unable because of pulmonary disease or muscle weakness to clear the lungs.
4. Compromised immune system: Immunocompromised patients are especially vulnerable to infection. Therefore, aggressive medical care is critical. Calculating a risk-benefit ratio regarding oral nutrition and hydration is equally critical. Aggressive rehabilitation, assuming the patient's health and mentation permit, altered diets, and admittedly costly feeding preparation and feeding programs may preserve health and quality of life in the long run. They may even be most cost-effective than nonoral nutrition.

Combining the variables and their mechanism of influence on health gives rise to a number of specific treatment planning guidelines.

1. A clinician can work out a rough likelihood of a patient's getting ill by tabulating the number of risks. For example, an aspirating patient who is otherwise independent and in good health has a lower chance of illness than does one who is confined to the bed and is dependent on others for feeding and oral care. Risks attend this use of the data, of course, because it treats all of them more or less equally. Nonetheless, the risks can be balanced by the benefit of being appropriately but humbly aggressive or conservative as one's clinical judgment dictates.
2. Presence of these variables dictates an aggressive program of rehabilitation if the patient can tolerate it and if consistent with the overall plan for medical/surgical management.
3. The type of treatment may be indicated by these variables. Aggressive oral hygiene is indicated in those with risk of colonization. Expiratory muscle strength training (EMST) may be recommended for those with poor pulmonary clearance, and so on.
4. Aggressive compensatory approaches can also be motivated by these data and by the recognition that aspirators will aspirate. As tube feeding does not prevent aspiration, but rather only what is aspirated, clinicians can complete a cost-benefit ratio for initiating oral intake in patients with dysphagia. What is to be balanced, unless the patient has already announced a decision about oral or nonoral nutrition, is presumed health status and quality of life. In general, quality of life can be threatened by nonoral nutrition and even by altered diets, especially if they involve pureed foods and thickened liquids. Therefore, the most normal diet, the safest posture for eating and drinking, the safest bolus size and rate of eating or drinking, intensive monitoring and even feeding, aggressive oral hygiene, and attention to health status may often keep someone eating.
5. The point to recall is this: both oral and nonoral nutrition have risks. Choosing among those risks is the responsibility of health care teams working with patients and families.

These data on likelihood of illness have limitations. First, the subjects were all veterans being served in VA facilities; therefore, the data may not apply to general populations of dysphagic persons or to those with movement disorders. A second limitation to the data for planning purposes is the absence of a method of analysis to create risk ratios for the variables alone or in combination. Nonetheless, they give clinicians concerned with avoiding patient illness from aspiration guidance about when to be more or less conservative. A third caveat is that the pneumonias occurring in these two groups of patients were not inevitably the result of prandial aspiration. In other words, it may well have been that reflux or infected oral materials carried into the lungs with aspirated saliva were the causes in many. This is important to recognize, because preventing aspiration pneumonia in such patients is not as simple as eliminating oral diets. Aspirators will aspirate. Finally, these data must be interpreted with considerable intellect. A reflexive interpretation might lead a clinician to mistakenly say that tubes are inappropriate because they are associated with illness. The issue is much more complex. A period of tube feeding to stabilize nutrition and hydration parameters, assuming the patient agrees, is absolutely appropriate in some cases. Tube feeding's presence on the list occurred because tube-fed patients are often restricted to their beds, dependent, confused, and otherwise seriously ill. These characteristics may be more critical than the presence of the tube. Nonetheless, these data have their uses.

REPORTING THE RESULTS

Chapter 8 contains the outline for a report of all data, including a section for the history. The relevant findings from the chart review and history are to be reported there. Their interpretation is best included in the assessment and discussion.

SUMMARY

The chart review and history contribute to treatment planning and set the stage for a subsequent clinical and perhaps instrumental assessment of the swallowing mechanism. These procedures may reveal the unexpected or may merely confirm expectations. They will also contribute to the clinician's understanding about the psychological and physiological reasons for the dysphagia. They will also contribute to treatment planning, sometimes by merely being confirmatory and sometimes by providing fresh insights into what should happen to help the patient.

5 Clinical Swallow Examination

The clinical swallow examination (CSE) is the heart of clinical practice. Attempts to relegate it to the status of screening examination are to be resisted. This examination sets the agenda for all else that happens between the patient and clinician. Its competent performance is the measure of a clinician's excellence.

EXPECTATIONS OF THE EXAMINATION

The CSE is the sophisticated clinician's most powerful tool. A maximum expectation of the procedure is that it will inform the perspicacious diagnostician about:

1. The likelihood that a person has a dysphagia
2. Selected signs, especially drooling, loss of bolus between the lips, reduced chewing, and even rocking of the bolus
3. The likelihood of penetration and aspiration with signs like wet voice, coughing, choking, and changes in breathing
4. Estimate of velopharyngeal function, realizing that velopharyngeal function in swallow will differ from that function in speech or upon observation of elevation during /a/
5. Estimate of laryngeal function with the same caveats
6. Determination of peripheral upper extremity mobility
7. Determination of cognitive status, including memory and attention
8. Insight into the patient's ability to perceive and manipulate food and drink and reaction to food and drink
9. With the right clinical manipulations, determination of what treatments are most likely to be effective
10. Other problems patient may have, such as poor dentition, that could influence evaluation or treatment
11. Whether or not an instrumental examination is necessary for further assessment

Caveat

Few, however, are the clinicians willing to grant this much power to the CSE. Typical complaints are that aspiration may be missed and that a physiologically oriented treatment cannot be derived. A clinical book is not the forum for a discussion of these issues. Rather, it is our position that in the right hands, the CSE is

25

a powerful tool and should not be reflexively supplanted by an instrumented examination. Done right, it has multiple possibilities for providing critical functional information that a necessarily brief videofluoroscopc swallow examination (VFSE) or a longer videoendoscopic swallow examination may not provide.

SPECIFIC PROCEDURES

Nowhere, perhaps, is clinical freedom more obvious than in the variety of clinical examinations for swallowing (and speech) disorders. The diversity probably reflects differences in training, differences in clinical environment, and what turn out to be the multiple reasons why a clinician might give a clinical examination to a person with dysphagia. One would hope that the literature could be a guide and perhaps it can. However, most of the data-based articles are devoted to identifying those clinical procedures that elicit responses (such as dysphonia) that are correlated with penetration and aspiration events. This is an important but narrow purpose. Therefore, what follows is an outline of the main components of a clinical examination, along with some typical tasks (or tests) and their interpretation.

General Observations

First contacts with a patient are informative. In dysphagia one wants specifically to note:

1. General alertness, orientation, and ability to attend
2. Physical ability such as ability to sit unsupported

3. Presence of rigidity, weakness, tremor, dystonia, and other movement abnormalities involving body and swallowing structures
4. Drooling
5. Presence of dysarthria, although it is to be remembered that speech and swallow can be differentially affected in neurologic and other disease
6. Presence of a tracheostomy
7. Presence of a feeding tube
8. Presence and use of suction
9. Ability to stand, transfer, walk
10. Ability to understand
11. Well- or ill-kept appearance
12. Cachexia
13. Mood
14. Dentition
15. Suspected or confirmed use of alcohol or tobacco
16. Difficulty breathing

Once these general observations have been made, the more formal part of the exam can begin.

Bulbar Sensory-Motor Examination

The usual purpose of this examination is to evaluate the various structures and movements critical to the oropharyngeal swallow and to derive a hypothesis about why they are abnormal when they are. It is important to note that *not all observations are equally important for all patients and some may be relatively trivial for the majority*. Nonetheless, this list of potential activities will be reasonably complete. It is for the individual clinician to decide if a particular task or interpretation is useful to the understanding of a particular patient's swallowing pattern. An outline of the examination is included in Table 5–1.

Table 5–1. The bulbar swallowing structures, selected tasks, and the interpretation of performance

Structure	Task	Interpretation
Lips/face	Seal against clinician movement, pucker, and smile Test response to touch bilaterally	Impairment may be part of explanation for drooling, failure to retain bolus in mouth, or pocketing of bolus after swallow
Tongue	Protrude, move laterally, resist clinician pressure against tongue in cheek Elevate tongue to hard palate with mouth open, produce /k/ without and then with a bite block in place A bite block can be easily accomplished by asking the patient to place the thumb laterally between the teeth to challenge lingual function in greater isolation Test response to touch bilaterally	The tongue is critical to swallowing, especially bolus formation and posterior movement; therefore, an impaired tongue may help explain poor bolus formation or inadequate propulsion of bolus into pharynx
Jaw	Lower and move jaw left and right against resistance while the clinician palpates masseter muscle function	May help to explain inefficient chewing
Hard palate and velum	Visual inspection of the velum with the patient producing /a/ has some value regarding velar movement Challenge velar function with an assimilative nasality task to listen for hypernasality: "Make me a Hong Kong cookie." Listen to connected speech for imbalances in resonance	Reduced palatal movement may aid interpretation of escape of bolus through nose and reduced propulsion of bolus into the pharynx
Larynx	Cough and *coup de glotte* (grunt) Palpation of hyolaryngeal movement with volitional and reflexive swallowing Production of /a/ to assess voice quality Pitch glide with /a/ from low to high Repeat /a/ several times quickly Listen to voice quality in connected speech	May suggest poor laryngeal valving during swallowing Need to remember that laryngeal valving for speech and swallow may be differentially involved
Respiratory mechanism	Sniff, pant, test of vocal loudness Maximum phonation duration with /a/ if appropriate Determine ability to roll over in bed and ability to sit unsupported Listen to loudness of connected speech	May implicate respiratory involvement in total dysphagia pattern

These special tests and observations can give the clinician an idea about structure integrity and movement. However, nothing is more important than actually watching a patient move a bolus to the mouth, prepare it for swallowing, and then swallow it.

Eating Examination/Trial Swallows

Trial swallows using liquids and foods are an important part of the CSE. Well-chosen procedures will give the perspicacious clinician insight into a swallowing problem in ways that the traditional clinical and instrumental examinations cannot. The procedures need not be standardized. Instead, the clinician needs to provide food and drink the patient or family report as being difficult and then make note of the patient's handling of these materials. Setting up the evaluation to resemble a meal is often the best policy. Depending on patient characteristics, letting the individual control the first part of the exam and the clinician the second can be valuable. For example, if a patient obviously is eating too rapidly and coughing, the clinician can replicate the boluses but control the rate to determine relative effects on coughing, choking, and other patient signs.

This eating examination can even yield quantifiable observations. One method that may be particularly helpful as a diagnostic and functional outcomes measure is to time the patient's consuming a specified amount of food or liquid. The interpretation may be complicated by upper extremity involvement, vision, desire, and a host of other influences. Nonetheless, experienced clinicians can derive valuable information.

The eating examination can reveal:

1. Patterns of difficulty such as poor ability to move food or drink to the mouth
2. Rapid or slow ingestion of food or drink
3. Order of food and drink
4. Bite and drink size
5. Distractibility
6. Failure to chew or swallow efficiently
7. Posture during eating
8. Chewing motion
9. Difficulty identifying food or drink
10. Difficulty locating the food or drink
11. Coughing, choking, throat clearing, and changes in breathing
12. Other problems that alone or in combination may explain a dysphagia

One further word on the trial swallows portion of the examination. It is important to remember that swallowing is a part of eating and that a swallowing deficit may be in part or in whole an eating deficit.

GENERAL YIELD OF THE CSE

The CSE will yield useful data only to the degree the examiner is systematic and observant. In the hands of such an examiner, the following may be revealed:

1. General signs and symptoms
2. Signs and symptoms of abnormal eating
3. Signs and symptoms of abnormal swallowing
4. Hypotheses, regardless of how tentative, about the possibility of penetration and aspiration

5. Hypotheses about the reasons for all signs and symptoms with emphasis, of course, upon the swallowing
6. Treatment ideas suggested by the examination
7. Specific recommendations for follow-up, including need for an instrumental examination, treatment, follow-up, or referral to another specialty

REPORTING THE RESULTS

The CSE allows the clinician to observe structure and movement integrity specific to those structures important in swallowing both during nonswallowing and swallowing tasks. In addition, each patient's general characteristics, such as appearance of health or illness, can be cataloged. Chapter 8 provides an outline for reporting these and all other findings.

CONCLUSIONS

When combined with the chart review and history, the CSE may be the only examination a patient needs. If not, the results can almost always direct the examiner to the next critical step in assessment. Chapter 6 contains a description of videofluoroscopy and Chapter 7 covers videoendoscopy. This order is not to be interpreted as a recommendation of test order or to rank the benefits of the various assessment procedures. That is determined by the patient's signs and the clinician's interpretation of them.

6 Videofluoroscopic Swallow Examination

The videofluoroscopic swallow examination (VFSE) requires the diagnostician to interpret shadows of structures and the interaction of these shadows with the barium bolus flow. Its usefulness is determined primarily by experience. Experience involves the tutored reading of hundreds of examinations, although the insightful person can begin to appreciate landmarks and patterns after 50 or so exams if the tutoring is thorough. Experience is best if it is also accompanied by the completion of several examinations per week and the careful reading of each. Careful reading means playing the examinations in a light-controlled room several times at normal and frame-by-frame speeds. Furthermore, the individual structures and movements of the swallowing mechanism and bolus need to be observed specifically, perhaps after the entire swallow has been viewed one or more times, to get a feeling for the overall patterns. Bolus preparation, including guaranteeing adequate density for easy interpretation, is also of critical importance and will be discussed more thoroughly below. The structure of the exam can only be specified generally, as different centers, clinicians, and purposes will determine the particulars. Nonetheless, certain general parameters can be outlined.

THE VIEW

A lateral view (see Figure 6–1) should capture the lips anteriorly and the spinal column posteriorly. In our experience, the anterior view of the oral stage is often neglected in comparison to imaging of pharyngeal and laryngeal swallowing events. This is something to be cautioned against, as assessment of oral stage function is critical to interpreting oropharyngeal biomechanics.

Superiorly, the soft palate should be captured and the bottom of the upper esophageal sphincter (UES; C-7 as a minimum) inferiorly. Patient alignment is also critical and one way of judging this is to observe the mandible. The best alignment is signaled by a single outline of the ramus rather than the appearance of both rami.

An anterior-posterior (A-P) view (see Figure 6–2) can establish symmetry of bolus flow through the pharynx and UES. The A-P view can also be filmed with the person standing so that the esophagus can be scanned. However, such scanning does not constitute formal assessment of esophageal function as may be obtained with an esophogram or barium swallow. If esophageal motility

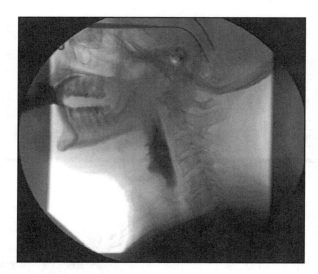

Figure 6–1. Lateral view of the swallow during the videofluoroscopic swallow exam (VFSE). From "Dysphagia in Patients with Motor Speech Disorders," by J. C. Rosenbek and H. N. Jones, 2006, in G. Weismer (Ed.), *Motor Speech Disorders* (p. 227), San Diego, CA: Plural Publishing. Reprinted with permission.

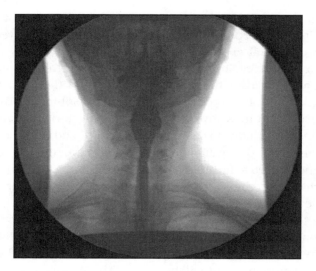

Figure 6–2. Anterior-posterior (A-P) view of the swallow during the videofluoroscopic swallow exam. From "Dysphagia in Patients with Motor Speech Disorders," by J. C. Rosenbek and H. N. Jones, 2006, in G. Weismer (Ed.), *Motor Speech Disorders* (p. 227), San Diego, CA: Plural Publishing. Reprinted with permission.

or obstruction is suspected, recommendation of referral to a radiologist or gastroenterologist is mandatory.

For clinicians using the Penetration-Aspiration Scale (PAS; Rosenbek, Robbins, Roecker, Coyle, & Wood, 1996), it is critical to continue imaging for at least 2 seconds after each swallow to allow for the most reliable scoring of response to penetration and aspiration. For more details on the PAS, see further discussion below and Appendix B.

THE BOLUSES

Generally, boluses should vary in viscosity and type. They must be sufficiently opaque to allow easy interpretation of bolus flow. Thin and thick boluses are traditional and commercial products can be employed to standardize the varieties of both thin and thick. In our experience, these commercial products may also ensure sufficient opacity to improve a clinician's ability to interpret the exam.

Solid boluses at a minimum should include one or more cookie pieces in barium. Barium tablets can also be used to approximate pill swallowing. Real foods coated in barium may also be useful. Bolus amounts can vary and probably should in most cases:

- Small (less than 5 ml) boluses may underestimate true swallowing performance but are often preferred as a starting place to control aspiration of large amounts.
- Boluses between 10 and 20 ml approximate the sizes persons normally consume. The clinician needs to decide in every case what

is appropriate. In some instances, larger boluses may result in improved swallowing.

- A reasonably safe scheme is to start with smaller and move to larger boluses.
- Large, serial swallows are nearly always informative but require a mature clinician capable of judging the dividend of these potentially more challenging boluses. A rule is that small boluses are more likely to be safer, and larger, more natural boluses are more likely to be informative.
- The bolus size for solids is less standardized. About the only published guideline is one fourth of a small cookie coated with barium paste (Logemann, 1983). Bolus size for solids is also up to the clinician, although new commercial products are under development that provide solid boluses in ¼- and ½-inch sizes.

Various centers also have a variety of diets (e.g., soft mechanical). Although these are not generally standard across institutions, an individual clinician can choose to test one or more of what is standard in the center or community.

METHOD OF ADMINISTRATION

Swallowing performance can be influenced by how boluses are delivered. However, specific effects are difficult to predict with precision. Nonetheless, we advocate both clinician and patient administered boluses for diagnostic and functional purposes.

Clinician administered boluses with the clinician also determining when the patient is to swallow are the norm. The control can be informative and most likely has diagnostic significance. This method of administration also allows the clinician to retain control over the exam, which may be valuable in terms of safety in some cases, such as when aspiration is of particular concern or when patients suffer from impulsivity.

Patient control of bolus amounts and of the timing of the initiation of the swallow is likely to have more functional significance. Additionally, this is more likely to reflect performance outside of the fluoroscopy suite. Providing patients with the various delivery devices they may commonly encounter (e.g., cup, straw, spoon) is also appropriate for the clinician using the examination to assess functional (as opposed to diagnostic) status.

SPECIAL MANIPULATIONS

The best VFSE is not only diagnostic but also provides functional data and information for treatment planning. These gains are realized, however, only by clinicians employing a variety of postural and therapeutic maneuvers during VFSE. Special manipulations can be considered as a drop-down menu of options tailored to individuals based on a variety of factors such as cognitive-linguistic status, swallowing signs, and overall health status.

The simplest manipulations are postural adjustments. The first is the chin tuck, with the amount of tuck determined for the individual. Another is the head turn, with our recommendation that turning both left and right is the best procedure,

as side of maximum deficit is harder to predict in movement disorders than in stroke, for example. Head turns can also vary in severity. If bolus flow is only passing down one side, repeating a swallow with the head turned to that side can alert the diagnostician to the possibility that passage down the other side is blocked, perhaps by a tumor or weakness. Combining the chin tuck and head turn may also pay dividends. Bracing the patient's head by whatever means available can also be useful, although this is typically easier during the clinical swallow exam (CSE) than during the VFSE, unless one uses a special chair with head support.

Planned treatment procedures, such as some of those encountered in Chapter 13 and Chapter 14, can also be tested at least to some degree during the VFSE. Realistically, this requires more time and the cooperation of the often multiple disciplines present at a VFSE. The most economical way to proceed is for the clinician to anticipate what methods may make sense clinically and then train the patient prior to the examination so that a team does not have to wait while a person is learning the supraglottic swallow or some other procedure. Procedures to try with adequate advanced patient training include:

1. Hard swallow in its various permutations
2. Mendelsohn maneuver
3. Supraglottic swallow
4. The variety of sensory stimulation modalities, including temperature, sour, and electrical
5. Unless the therapeutic effect is spectacular, skill is required in deciding how many swallows of a particular sort are required for a conclusion about the possible helpfulness of

a posture or technique. Generally, clinicians are left with only modest confidence about the effect of a particular swallowing adaptation. However, these impressions can then be confirmed in follow-up visits.

READING THE EXAMINATION

We know that reading or interpretation mistakes are diminished in proportion to the number of examinations a clinician has done and the quality of original and continued training. Other factors can also influence the interpretation, such as patient posture during the examination, the density of the barium preparation, preexisting structural anomalies, patient cooperation, and patient movement during the examination.

We recommend reading all films in a dark room after the examination is complete. The VFSE requires the interpretation of shadows. Bright light in the reading room may obscure these shadows. We recommend viewing the examination several times at normal speed and then frame by frame, as needed. We also recommend enough repetitions so that one can focus on individual structures in relationship to bolus flow. So, for example, on one viewing the velum can be the focus of attention, the larynx on another, the UES on another, and so on. Too often in modern clinical practice, the larynx is the focus of the examination. This may limit the utility of the exam.

Using the PAS (see Appendix B) requires looking at the density of all shadows to determine what densities are present before barium is offered so as to make decisions about the occurrence of penetration and aspiration and whether material is expelled from the airway.

Most clinicians using the VFSE in clinical practice do not make sophisticated durational measures, although using a timer is standard in some centers and relatively easy to introduce if a facility wishes to. Leonard and Kendall (2007) is a good resource for further information about durational measures in dysphagia assessment.

Several checklists have been published that allow the clinician to systematically report presence or absence of a variety of dysphagia signs. A sample from our own work is included in Table 6–1.

A checklist is not comfortable for some practitioners, who prefer to describe signs according to their training and perhaps requirements for report format particular to their institution. As a minimum, the complete report, however, can profitably include the following:

1. Observations on the integrity of swallow structures.
2. Observations on the relationship of swallow structure movements to bolus movement. For example, the position of the bolus when the hyoid starts its final upward and forward movement, the position of the bolus when laryngeal closure occurs, and when UES opening begins are all potentially important observations.
3. Observations about timing (Lof & Robbins, 1990), completeness, and direction of bolus flow are also traditional and can be helpful as shown in Table 6–1. For example, the two most important directional measures are penetration (see Figure 6–3) and aspiration (See Figure 6–4) in which material is misdirected into the airway.

Table 6–1. A checklist of major bolus flow abnormalities that can be extracted from the VFSE.

Abnormality	How Measured
Durational Measures	
Duration of oral transit	Time from initiation of posterior movement of bolus to time of arrival of bolus head at ramus of mandible
Duration of stage transition	Time from arrival of bolus head at ramus to time at beginning of hyolaryngeal complex elevation
Duration of pharyngeal transit	Time from head of bolus first reaching posterior border of mandibular ramus to tail of bolus exiting UES
Duration of UES opening	Time from bolus arrival at leading margin of UES to time tail of bolus exits the UES
Duration of laryngeal closure	Time from first closure of larynx during swallow to time of beginning abduction
Duration of total swallow	Time from initiation of posterior bolus flow in mouth to time of tail of bolus exiting the UES
Duration of velar closure	Time from first contact of velum and posterior pharyngeal wall to time that contact is broken
Stasis	
Oral stasis	Slight, mild, moderate, severe, profound
Pharyngeal stasis	Slight, mild, moderate, severe, profound
Vallecular stasis	Slight, mild, moderate, severe, profound
Pyriform sinus stasis	Slight, mild, moderate, severe, profound
Misdirection	
Penetration of larynx	Scores 2 through 5 of the PAS
Aspiration	Scores 6 through 8 of the PAS
Nasal regurgitation	Slight, mild, moderate, severe, profound

INTERPRETATION OF THE DATA

The VFSE contributes data to the management of those with movement disorders. The critical notion, however, is that these data are but one part of the data bank necessary to management. This point is reiterated here because the virtues of the VFSE have been oversold in much traditional and even contemporary writing. Contributions to the following, however, can be expected.

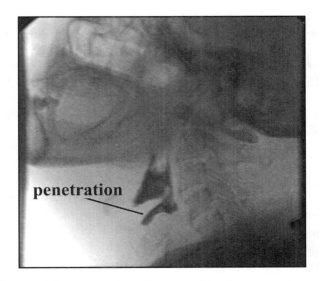

Figure 6–3. Penetration during a videofluoroscopic swallow examination. From "Dysphagia in Patients with Motor Speech Disorders," by J. C. Rosenbek and H. N. Jones, 2006, in G. Weismer (Ed.), *Motor Speech Disorders* [plate 9], San Diego, CA: Plural Publishing. Reprinted with permission.

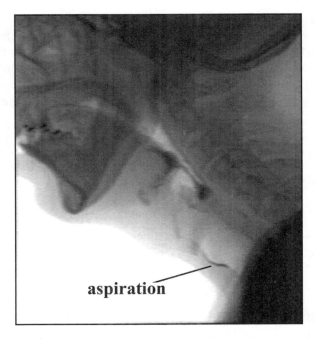

Figure 6–4. Aspiration during a videofluoroscopic swallow examination. From "Dysphagia in Patients with Motor Speech Disorders," by J. C. Rosenbek and H. N. Jones, 2006, in G. Weismer (Ed.), *Motor Speech Disorders* [plate 11], San Diego, CA: Plural Publishing. Reprinted with permission.

Presence or Absence of Dysphagia

Judgments can be aided concerning the presence or absence of dysphagia. No universally agreed-upon set of signs signals the presence of dysphagia, however. Clinicians are left to make judgments about how slowness, stasis, and bolus misdirection are to be interpreted. This means that some patients may be identified as having dysphagia by some clinicians and as normal by others.

Dysphagia in some patients, of course, is obvious, as when aspiration occurs on multiple swallows or when the UES opening is so reduced as to permit only minimal bolus passage, even with consecutive swallows. In others, the decision is harder and requires appeals to clinical experience. That is, the longer one has been examining patients, the more likely it is that a distribution of normal and abnormal swallows is stored in the clinician's brain. Balancing of patient and family report with the results of the VFSE should also be done, and this too is a skill that improves with experience.

Establishing Signs of the Dysphagia

This can be done by considering durational measures, stasis, and misdirected bolus flow (see Table 6–1).

Identifying Structural or Physiologic Abnormalities

The VSFE can help in identifying the structural or physiologic abnormalities that may contribute to the dysphagia. Patients with movement disorders may also have osteophytes, Zenker's diverticulum, and even head and neck cancers. Therefore, it is critical for the clinician to read each examination with an unbiased eye, as medical conditions associated with dysphagia may be superimposed on one another.

Bolus flow may be too fast or too slow, although slowness must be conservatively judged because "slowness" in older patients may be adaptive.

Bolus propulsion may be inadequate, a condition often assumed to reflect weakness of swallowing musculature. It is important to remember that the exact influences of weakness and abnormal tone have never been proven in any neurologic disorder. Therefore, the careful clinician talks about strength and tone abnormalities as hypothesized rather than confirmed.

Incoordination of swallowing structure movements is frequent in patients with movement disorders. For example, boluses may arrive at the UES before it has opened sufficiently or into the pharynx before laryngeal closure has occurred, and so on.

Identifying the Presence of Penetration and Aspiration

The most serious bolus flow abnormalities are penetration and aspiration. We use the PAS (Rosenbek, Robbins, et al., 1996) to quantify these abnormalities. The PAS is a psychometrically-sound, eight-point, equal-appearing scale. It appears in Appendix B. The two major dimensions scored are depth of passage of material into the airway and the patient's reaction to these events. Score 1 is assigned if the bolus does not enter the airway. Scores 2, 3, 4, and 5 are assigned depending on depth of penetration into the larynx and whether or not patient successfully ejects this material. Scores 6, 7, and 8 are assigned to episodes of aspiration and whether or not the patient effectively responds. Scores of 1, 2, and 3 are often seen in normal swallowers of all ages, especially in older adults. No single occurrence of any score determines a person's normality or abnormality. Referral sources usually are more concerned with penetration and aspiration than with any other sign, so quantification of it can be helpful.

Establishing the Influence of Treatment Techniques on Swallowing Biomechanics

An experienced clinician can get at least some idea about the influence of posture and even some rehabilitative techniques on swallowing performance. Usually it is most efficient to instruct the patient prior to initiating the VFSE. The challenge is in knowing how many repetitions of any manipulation to try before concluding it may or may not be helpful. This number cannot be dictated and must be guided by clinical experience. The safest procedure is to follow up clinically with any promising procedure, because a safe swallow in the test suite may disappear with multiple swallows, other bolus types, distractions, and so on.

Determining the Need for Compensations

This includes decisions about whether or not an individual is appropriate for an oral diet or not. This decision is challenging and it is our view that the VFSE should never be the only guide to recommending recommending an oral diet or any other treatment decision. The VFSE can, however, give the clinician some idea about the proper bolus type, size, administration technique, the need for assistance with meals, and other similar information. Clinical follow-up in natural environments whenever possible is critical. Recommending that a patient and family maintain a swallowing diary, for example, may be valuable.

REPORTING THE DATA

All of these findings are to be reported. In general, the more quantification, the better. However, most referral sources want to know the implications as well. The implications about the structural and physiologic explanations for the bolus flow abnormalities can be included as well as hypotheses. The implications for treatment planning, type of diet, and the rest depend on an integration of all data, including that from the chart review, history, CSE, and VFSE. Therefore, a separate chapter (Chapter 8) devoted exclusively to the report is included in this volume.

SUMMARY

The VFSE provides important data for the assessment and treatment of swallowing disorders in patients with movement disorders. In our opinion, it is usually the best swallow examination in this population because it enhances the chance of directly observing the movement abnormalities that contribute to the dysphagia. Other issues of planning require the data to be collated with data from all other procedures.

7 Videoendoscopic Swallow Examination

The videoendoscopic swallow examination, often referred to as the *fiberoptic endoscopic evaluation of swallowing* (FEES®), was first described by Langmore, Schatz, and Olsen in 1988. Videoendoscopy allows the dysphagia clinician to directly visualize the pharyngeal and laryngeal structures and their performance before and after the swallow. This is accomplished via transnasal passage of a flexible endoscope into the pharynx, as shown Figure 7–1 and Figure 7–2. Much like the videofluoroscopic swallow examination (VFSE), the usefulness of this approach to assess swallowing is determined primarily by experience. What follows is a general overview of the exam, though we acknowledge that different centers, clinicians, and purposes will determine the particulars.

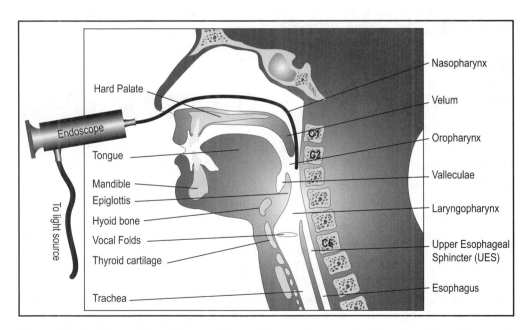

Figure 7–1. Illustration of the position of the endoscope during the videoendoscopic swallow examination.

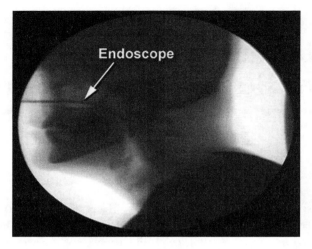

Figure 7–2. Position of the endoscope during the videoendoscopic swallow examination as seen with fluoroscopy. From *"Understanding Dysphagia"* (Version 1.0) [CD], by J. Murray and N. Musson, 2005, Department of Veterans Affairs, Veteran Health Administration. Reprinted with permission.

THE VIEW

Videoendoscopy provides a superior view of pharyngeal and laryngeal structures, as seen in Figure 7–3 and Figure 7–4. The view comprises the pharyngeal wall posteriorly and the vallecular space anteriorly. Laterally, the left and right pyriform sinuses should be visualized. The endoscope is passed transnasally into the pharynx to a position just above the epiglottis.

Videoendoscopy does not allow for visualization of the oral structures or their function during swallowing. During the swallow, a period of "whiteout" occurs at the phase of pharyngeal contraction. In this short period of time, the view is obscured for 300 to 500 milliseconds (Aviv & Murry, 2005; Perlman & Van Deale, 1993). Swallowing performance is assessed based on visualization of pharyngeal and laryngeal structures before and after the swallow.

THE BOLUSES

In some centers, a topical anesthetic and/or decongestant is sprayed into the nasal passage prior to introduction of the endoscope. We typically find this not to be necessary and that lubricating the scope to reduce friction is sufficient for patient comfort.

Prior to bolus administration, pharyngeal and laryngeal structures should be observed. For example, laryngeal integrity with phonation and cough is assessed. Determination of the presence of secretions, as well as their severity and location,

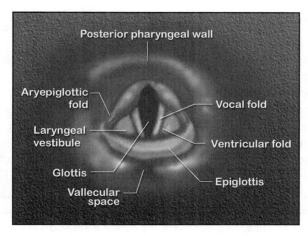

Figure 7–3. Illustration of pharyngeal and laryngeal structures as visualized during the videoendoscopic swallow examination. From "*Understanding Dysphagia*" (Version 1.0) [CD], by J. Murray and N. Musson, 2005, Department of Veterans Affairs, Veteran Health Administration. Reprinted with permission.

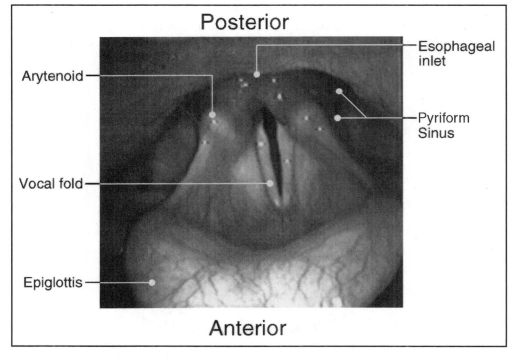

Figure 7–4. Pharyngeal/laryngeal appearance as visualized during the videoendoscopic swallow examination. From "*FEEST: Flexible Endoscopic Evaluation of Swallowing with Sensory Testing*" (p 9.), by J. E. Aviv and T. Murry, 2005, San Diego, CA: Plural Publishing. Reprinted with permission.

should be completed. Assessment of secretion management is a valuable contribution of videoendoscopic exam. An example of laryngeal secretions is seen in Figure 7–5.

If sensory testing is to be completed, it is recommended this be done prior to any bolus administrations. For more information on sensory testing or *flexible endoscopic evaluation of swallowing with sensory testing* (FEESST), see Aviv and Murry (2005) and Aviv et al. (1998).

Unlike the VFSE, videoendoscopy does not require ingestion of radiopaque barium boluses. Rather, it is common to use regular food and drink that has been dyed blue or green to contrast with the colors of the pharynx and larynx. However, some clinicians prefer to use food and liquids without dye, and this has been reported to result in reliable results (Leder, Acton, Lisitano, & Murray, 2005).

Generally, boluses should vary in viscosity and type. Thin and thick liquid boluses are traditional, and commercial products can be employed to standardize the varieties of thick liquids. Solid boluses should include, at a minimum, pudding and cookie swallows. Other foods may also be useful, especially if they are reported to be problematic for a particular individual. Bolus amounts can and probably should vary in most cases. The discussion of bolus sizes in Chapter 6 is also appropriate for videoendoscopy.

METHOD OF ADMINISTRATION

As with VFSE, swallowing performance can be influenced by how boluses are delivered, though specific effects are dif-

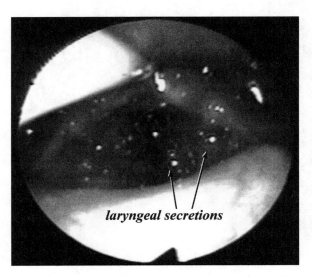

laryngeal secretions

Figure 7–5. Secretions visualized during the video-endoscopic swallow examination. From "Dysphagia in Patients with Motor Speech Disorders," by J. C. Rosenbek and H. N. Jones, 2006, in G. Weismer (Ed.), *Motor Speech Disorders* [plate 8], San Diego, CA: Plural Publishing. Reprinted with permission.

ficult to predict with precision. Nonetheless, we advocate both clinician and patient administered boluses for diagnostic and functional purposes. Boluses administered by a third party (a trained assistant is best) under the direction of the clinician are the norm. The clinician is unable to directly administer boluses due to the need to hold and control the endoscope. However, the clinician retains control over the administration of boluses and may have the patient swallow on command.

Patient controlled bolus amounts and timing of the initiation of the swallow are likely to have more functional significance and reflect performance outside of the exam room. Using the various food and liquid delivery devices commonly encountered (e.g., cup, straw, spoon) is also appropriate.

SPECIAL MANIPULATIONS

The best videoendoscopic swallow exam provides functional data and information for treatment planning in addition to diagnostic information. Chapter 13 and Chapter 14 provide specific information about compensations and rehabilitation techniques that may be useful, depending on the swallowing signs. Additional considerations include the following.

Compared to VFSE, the duration of the exam can often be increased during videoendoscopy. Reasons for this include the fact that the procedure is generally under the more direct control of the dysphagia clinician and the lack of associated radiation exposure. This increased duration may be valuable to:

1. Determine the effects of fatigue on the swallow

2. Determine swallow function over a period of time that more closely approximates the duration of a normal meal
3. Allow more time to determine the effect of compensation and rehabilitation techniques on the swallow
4. Allow more time to elicit repeated swallows using compensation and rehabilitation techniques to more fully explore their value

In some cases, videoendoscopy can be used as a form of biofeedback to improve swallow performance. For example, the amount of effort required to close the airway with a forceful breath hold, such as with the supraglottic swallow (p. 99) or the Showa maneuver (p. 103), may be visualized by both the patient and the clinician.

READING THE EXAMINATION

As discussed in the previous chapter on VFSE, interpretation of exams improves based on experience and training. Other factors can also influence the interpretation, such as patient posture, cooperation, and movement during the exam, as well as structural abnormalities or secretions obfuscating the view.

We recommend viewing the examination several times at normal speed and then frame by frame as needed. It is important for the clinician to interpret the exam without the physical demands of performing endoscopy, especially when its duration is extended, so that full attention to the swallow can be marshaled. We also recommend enough repetitions so that one can focus on individual structures in relationship to bolus flow.

Consistent with our own experience, data from Kelly et al. (2007) suggest that videoendoscopy results in higher (i.e., more severe) PAS scores than does VFSE when the same swallows are scored. Kelly and colleagues (2006) also report that pharyngeal residue is rated to be more severe during the videoendoscopic exam in comparison to VFSE.

INTERPRETATION OF THE DATA

The videoendoscopic swallow exam contributes data to the management of those with movement disorders, though these data are but one part of the data bank necessary to management. Contributions to the following, however, can be expected.

Judging Presence or Absence of Dysphagia

There is no universally agreed-upon set of signs that signal the presence of dysphagia. Clinicians are left to make judgments about how stasis or bolus misdirection, for example, is to be interpreted. Dysphagia in some patients, of course, is obvious, such as when aspiration occurs on multiple swallows. In others, the decision is harder and requires appeals to clinical experience.

Establishing Signs of the Dysphagia

Aviv and Murry (2005) suggest use of the following terminology to describe pharyngeal and laryngeal abnormalities visualized during videoendoscopy:

1. Spillage, which occurs when a bolus enters the pharynx more than 1 second before the swallow
2. Pharyngeal residue
3. Penetration, or entry of material into the larynx above the level of the true vocal folds
4. Aspiration, or entry of material past the level of the true vocal folds
5. Reflux, or "the passage of material from the esophageal inlet retrograde into the laryngopharynx before, during, or after the swallow" (p. 39)

Use of the Penetration-Aspiration Scale (PAS; Rosenbek, Robbins, Roecker, Coyle, & Wood, 1996; see Appendix B) during videoendoscopy has been described in the literature (Colodny, 2002; Kelly, Drinnan, & Leslie, 2007). For more details regarding the PAS, see the discussion in Chapter 6.

The presence of secretions, including severity and location, should be noted and is a critical contribution to the videoendoscopic exam.

Establishing Pharyngeal and Laryngeal Abnormalities

Establishing pharyngeal and laryngeal abnormalities may contribute to the dysphagia, and they include:

1. Overall, compared to the VFSE, we often find the videoendoscopic exam provides an improved view of the swallowing structures, particularly the pharynx and larynx. Examples of this follow below.
2. Vocal fold paralysis or paresis.
3. Evidence of pharyngeal and/or laryngeal trauma, such as ulceration or edema associated with prolonged or traumatic intubation.

4. Evidence suggesting possible gastroesophageal reflux disease (GERD), such as arytenoid/interarytenoid edema or erythema. For more details on this topic, we recommend Aviv and Murry's (2005) comprehensive discussion.

5. Other structural anomalies such as tumor. Although this may be unexpected in patients with movement disorders, medical conditions associated with dysphagia may be superimposed on one another, and it is therefore critical for the clinician to read each examination with an unbiased eye. We have even visualized severe osteophytes protruding from the posterior pharyngeal wall during videoendoscopy on one occasion.

6. When laryngeal involvement is greater than commonly encountered in a particular condition. For example, although in patients with PD dysphonia is commonly encountered and in fact expected, some patients present with dysphonia of greater severity than expected.

7. The videoendoscopic exam may also assist the dysphagia clinician in the determination of whether an individual has a single movement disorder or whether their difficulties are related to the presence of more than one movement disorder, such as when a patient has both PD and dystonia.

Establishing the Influence of Treatment Techniques on Swallowing Biomechanics

An experienced clinician can get at least some idea about the influence of compensatory and rehabilitative approaches on swallowing performance during the endoscopic exam. Although time constraints may be less rigid during videoendoscopy than during VFSE, it is usually prudent to instruct the patient prior to initiating the exam, especially with more complex techniques such as the supraglottic swallow. As always, the challenge is in knowing how many repetitions of any manipulation to try before concluding it may or may not be helpful. This number cannot be dictated and must be guided by clinical experience. We suggest the best practice is to follow up clinically with any promising procedure, because a safe swallow during the exam may disappear in natural environments.

Determining the Need for Compensations

This includes decisions about whether or not an individual is appropriate for an oral diet. This decision is challenging and it is our view that the endoscopic exam should never be the only guide to recommending or not recommending an oral diet or any other treatment decision. However, data from videoendoscopy, when combined with information from the history and chart review as well as other swallowing assessments such as the clinical swallow exam (CSE), can provide guidance in these decisions. Clinical follow-up in natural environments whenever possible is critical.

REPORTING THE DATA

All of these findings are to be reported. However, most referral sources want to know the implications of the findings as well. Implications for treatment planning, diet recommendations, and other such details depend on integration of all other available data, which at a minimum should include information from the chart review and history, as well as the CSE and VFSE in some cases. A separate chapter (Chapter 8) devoted exclusively to the report is included in this volume.

CAVEAT

Most contemporary authors (Langmore, 2003) suggest that videofluoroscopy and videoendoscopy are complementary, rather than competing, procedures for swallow assessment, and this is certainly consistent with our own clinical experience. However, in our clinical practices with patients with movement disorders, we most commonly employ VFSE when an instrumental exam is indicated. A primary reason for this is the prominence of oral stage deficits in those with movement disorders, especially those with parkinsonian features. Instances when videoendoscopy may be preferred have been discussed above and will be further discussed in the forthcoming chapters on specific patient populations.

SUMMARY

The videoendoscopic swallow examination provides important data for the assessment and treatment of swallowing disorders in patients with dysphagia, including those with movement disorders.

8 The Report

Variability appropriately exists in the form of reports clinicians prepare, but usually in the particulars rather than in outline. However, even the outline will be determined in part by environmental influences, such as the requirements of the institution and third-party payers. Thus, dictating the shape and content of a report is treacherous business. Nonetheless, we will provide some general principles and our own organization to allow readers to compare their own practices to ours. We conceptualize the report as a document with three primary audiences: the referral source, dysphagia clinicians, and insurance providers and the institutions where the swallowing exam(s) is completed. Admittedly, there is a great deal of overlap in the information these primary audiences are interested in.

REFERRAL SOURCE

The report should be created with an eye toward the needs of the professional, usually a physician in the United States, who originally referred the patient. In other words, the report can provide answers to the questions asked in the consult along with some statement about the clinician's

confidence in those answers. For example, if the question is, "Does this patient aspirate?" providing an answer to that question will secure the referral source's good will and continued consultation. Of course, clinicians recognize that aspiration can be a complex phenomenon dependent on a host of variables such as attention, bolus type and size, fatigue, and the list goes on. Therefore, the clinician is usually left to provide a limited answer: "No aspiration observed on this examination," followed by an experience-based assessment of how likely that absence is to occur in the patient's life outside the VFSE suite.

Next, the clinician can provide other helpful information the referral source can benefit from but may not have known to ask about. This information may include:

1. Signs of the dysphagia as revealed by the clinical swallowing exam (CSE) and the instrumental examination(s).
2. Symptom status as revealed by history and SWAL-QOL.
3. Special influences on the dysphagia, such as responses to compensatory and rehabilitative methods tested during the clinical and instrumental examinations.

4. How likely an aspirator is to get sick from aspiration. These likelihoods have not been established for movement disorders, but Langmore and colleagues (1998) provide more general data on the variables associated with illness from aspiration that have been reported (see Chapter 4, including Table 4–2)

5. What the likely course of the dysphagia has been and will be—judgments, especially in the case of future course, that are usually reliant on a clinician's experience.

6. Patterns in the dysphagia, such as relationship to fatigue, poor sleep, emotional upset, time of day, medications, type of food and drink, and the like. Such patterns may inform the referring individual about medication and other adjustments to improve the swallow

7. Available behavioral treatments, expected outcomes, and intensity and duration of treatment. This section is especially important unless the consultant is very familiar with swallowing treatments.

8. Whether or not the pattern of swallowing performance is typical of the presumed medical diagnosis. In patients with movement disorders, this judgment can be difficult because of the relative dearth of data on patterns across diagnoses. Nonetheless, the experienced clinician with an active clinic can make reasonable statements in many cases. Medical diagnosis may also direct dysphagia clinicians toward reasonable ideas about treatment planning based on the presumed underlying neuromotor deficits and other factors. See the individual disorder chapters for more details.

DYSPHAGIA CLINICIANS

The report should also assist other dysphagia clinicians, usually speech-language pathologists (SLPs) in the United States, in understanding an individual's swallowing function at that moment. It is our view that quantification of observations is helpful, especially in an environment where SLPs are regarded as technicians rather than as independent practitioners. The usual form of quantification is a set of bolus flow abnormalities usually based on VFSE (see Table 6–1). In our movement disorders practice, an interdisciplinary clinic supported by a centralized data base, we report the following simplified set of numerical observations.

Severity of oral stage deficit reported on a five-point, equal-appearing interval scale with 0 being assigned to normal function and 4 being assigned to profound deficits. Descriptions accompany the number and commonly include mention of the adequacy of bolus control by the lips and tongue, slowness of movement, anterior to posterior bolus movement, postswallow oral residue, premature spillage of the bolus, and similar observations.

Severity of pharyngeal stage deficit is scored similarly. Descriptive statements may include amount and locus of residue, asymmetry if present, slowness of movement, and the presence when appropriate of structural abnormalities such as Zenker's diverticulum and cervical osteophytes on the cervical vertebrae. We also generally include the UES as part of this stage, but this may be a bit imprecise.

Worst score on the Penetration-Aspiration Scale (PAS; Rosenbek et al., 1998) gives an indication of laryngeal adequacy for swallowing (see Appendix B). Additional description regarding laryngeal events may also be necessary such as the timing, frequency, and amount of penetration and/or aspiration, the adequacy of hyolaryngeal movements, and so on.

All these scores are reliably assigned in our clinic because of our team's having worked together to achieve reliability. The same can occur in other clinics if scoring sessions are scheduled where the purpose is the reading of films and deriving scores by consensus. Our scoring is based on the presence of bolus flow and timing abnormalities and the clinician's assessment of their importance to the patient's complaint of swallowing problems. The scores function as a shorthand and are supplemented by the highlighting of important features of the swallow not necessarily captured by the scoring. For example, a cough or throat clear may be strong or weak or absent and immediate or delayed.

THIRD-PARTY PAYER/ INSTITUTIONAL EXPECTATIONS

In the United States, the report must also be written for the third-party payer and according to the requirements and expectations of the institution where the exam(s) occurred. This need not be a burden, as the required components are, for the most part, also components of thoughtful care. The components required in our practice appear below. It is important to recognize that not all payers require similar components, though Medicare sets the standard for the industry in adult patients. This list is not necessarily exhaustive, nor will all parts be necessary for all practitioners, especially considering different institutions may have different interpretations of what is required. The following list is provided as a sample for those who value specific suggestions:

1. Identifying information
2. Date of report
3. Date of examination or visit
4. Type of report (e.g., CSE)
5. Patient's name
6. Date of birth
7. Medical identification number
8. Insurance number, when appropriate
9. Examiner's affiliation
10. Examiner's credentials (e.g., CCC-SLP in the United States)
11. Patient's medical diagnosis
12. Date of onset, preferably at least month and year
13. Number of visits from start of care
14. Patient's treatment diagnosis, which refers to the condition for which the person is being seen. Most frequently this is dysphagia, although dysarthria, dementia, aphasia, and other conditions may co-occur and be evaluated during the same visit.
15. Reason for referral. In the United States, these statements typically are descriptive (e.g., "Patient is reported to choke on liquids and have difficulty swallowing pills.") and are accompanied by a statement of the function and quality of life implications of the condition (e.g., "Patient has fear of swallowing and is non-compliant with medication prescription."). The aim is to establish the *medical necessity* of the visit.
16. Who the report should be sent to, such as the referring physician and other appropriate members of the medical team as formally permitted by the patient.

MEDICAL HISTORY

Clinicians differ widely in their completeness in this section. Special emphasis on the swallowing history is obviously a key component of the medical history. Certainly, the details of the medical and social history relevant to the presence of dysphagia and its management, including prognosis for change with treatment, should be included. In our experience, an extremely detailed medical history is often provided at the expense of the social history. The value of the social history is not to be neglected, as it provides a rich, valuable source of data, particularly when making treatment recommendations. The social history need not be lengthy, but it should provide some information regarding considerations such as an individual's living circumstances, support for treatment if treatment is considered, and the patient's background such as current employment or previous occupation, educational history, and general interests.

EVALUATION

This section begins with a listing and description, as appropriate, of the diagnostic procedures or tests provided, followed by a structured presentation of the findings from each. In our clinic the usual components are some mixture of the following:

1. CSE
2. Instrumental examination—VFSE or videoendoscopy (sometimes, in rare instances, both)
3. SWAL-QOL (see Appendix A)

4. Measure of apathy (e.g., Apathy Evaluation Scale—Marin, Biedrzycki, & Firinciogullari, 1991; see Appendix C)
5. Mini-mental status examination (Folstein, Folstein, & McHugh, 1975)

IMPRESSIONS

Here is the core of the report where the clinician makes diagnostic and therapeutic sense of the findings in an intellectual way. Clearly, this is an instance where all the audiences for the swallowing report are interested. To be featured, of course, is the answer to the question posed by the referring professional. Additionally, the impact of the results on the medical diagnosis and plan for treatment are to be emphasized, along with appropriate commentary on the posited pathophysiology of the biomechanical abnormalities, any unusual features, and the functional, quality of life influence. The possible benefit (or lack thereof in some cases) of behavioral interventions (i.e., dysphagia therapy) should be discussed, including specific treatment approaches. This may be especially true at a tertiary care center where patients often receive follow-up care closer to home. Finally, recommendations for follow-up referrals and examinations by the report writer or by other professionals can be useful to the entire treatment team.

PLAN

The content of the plan can vary greatly, depending especially on whether dysphagia therapy is recommended. Recommendations should be clearly stated, even if previously referred to elsewhere such as in the impressions section. In addition to treatment recommendations, the plan should state referral and/or examination recommendations to the referring provider, as well as recommended follow-up exams with the dysphagia clinician including reevaluation at a recommended interval.

For those to be enrolled in dysphagia therapy, the requirements are more numerous. Typically we include the following:

1. Description of the treatment to be employed
2. Planned frequency and length of sessions
3. Total duration of treatment
4. Long-term goal(s): Reimbursement and good practice dictate that this be a functional goal, such as return to normal diet or 90% reduction in coughing episodes during mealtime.
5. Short-term goals: These goals need to be important and measurable. Because legitimate goals are so numerous it seems unwise to mention examples. Experienced clinicians will know how to write them and can teach newer clinicians.

PROGNOSIS

Prognosis for swallowing change should be stated (improvement, decline, or relative stability). If treatment is being recommended, the prognosis of the treatment's benefit to an individual should be stated. Prognosis is usually discussed in terms of excellent, good, fair, poor, and, in some cases, unknown (especially when the medical diagnosis is unknown with surety).

HISTORY OF PREVIOUS TREATMENT

It is important to determine the time and type of previous treatment. Reasons are numerous and some are included here.

Previous treatment can influence response to the planned treatment. A previously successful treatment might well cast a halo effect over the new treatment, especially if it is similar to the previously successful one. If the treatment was unsuccessful, the influence may contaminate the new, at least in the beginning.

Regardless of the effect, knowing what a previous clinician has done will help the present clinician formulate a plan. Seldom would a clinician want to reinitiate a previously unsuccessful treatment.

Knowing a patient was previously treated may also help explain symptoms. Disease usually produces a fairly typical set of signs, and idiosyncratic signs are likely the result of a person's attempting to cope with the disease or the results of treatment.

PATIENT AND FAMILY GOALS OF TREATMENT

Knowing what the patient and family expect will help focus a clinician's treatment approach. Although one might have to approach such goals in what a patient might see as an indirect way, as in selecting a physiologic target such as UES duration and extent of UES opening when the patient wants to eat pork chops, nonetheless, knowing the patient's goals for treatment will at a minimum remind the clinician to talk about the relationship of what the clinician is doing to what the patient wants. Knowing this information may also explain noncompliance or withdrawing from treatment, if the patient feels no progress is being made toward his or her goal.

EDUCATION AND COUNSELING

Explanations and counseling are mandated in the United States, even if they did not constitute quality patient care. Generally, explanation comprises a description of the form in which the education and counseling were completed and the patient's/family's apparent understanding and agreement. The counseling is not easily summarized in a sentence, but it occurs naturally for good clinicians and is essential for optimal clinical care. The swallowing exam and its results and the recommendations generated, as well as the medical condition that mandated

the assessment, are all potential sources of anxiety or grief. The alert, thoughtful clinician recognizes these potentially negative emotions and tries to neutralize them. How this is done can be documented.

SUMMARY

A good report is an intellectual document. It describes and explains and does so in language that all other health care team members can understand and appreciate. Done right, it also guarantees that persons with appropriate insurance will receive the coverage they are entitled to and that the clinician's institution will not be subject to review and potential charges of fraud. The report, whether it is done well or poorly, sets the stage for all subsequent patient and clinician contacts, as well as relationships with other health care professionals, such as the referral source.

9 Classification of Treatments

Treatments can generally be divided into compensatory and rehabilitative approaches, although the boundary of these two is indistinct and some methods may be more one or the other or neither, depending on how they are applied. We have preserved the distinction because we think it focuses clinicians on a major issue in dysphagia management—*the possibility that too many clinicians limit themselves to compensatory approaches*. In our view, rehabilitation should be the primary aim of treatment, and compensatory methods should be part of the plan only in conjunction with rehabilitation or if rehabilitation fails or is impossible. For us the reason is simple. The brain learns to do what it is forced to do. A brain whose body is tube fed will devote its critical real estate to activities the body is still performing.

Compensatory techniques are aimed at an immediate influence on safety and adequacy of nutrition and hydration. They are applied when a person needs immediate help either in the absence of rehabilitative efforts or in addition to them, or when a person cannot be expected to complete or profit from rehabilitative efforts. Once a decision in favor of compensatory approaches is made, it remains to choose the right ones and to derive a sense of security that the approach will indeed support safe, adequate nutrition

(pleasurable is sometimes possible as well). These are not easy decisions, although it is our experience that many clinicians seem to behave as if they can be made almost reflexively. Safety and adequacy are difficult to judge because evidence for both evolves over time. It may take days or weeks for malnutrition or dehydration to emerge, and the same is true for respiratory illness related to aspiration of food or drink. Thus, the clinician is left to predict based on the results of clinical and instrumental examinations, history, and clinical judgment. Chapter 13 describes the major compensatory treatments available to the dysphagia clinician working with patients with movement disorders (and often other conditions as well).

Rehabilitative techniques are designed and applied to improve swallowing function. They do so by improving the skilled movements necessary to a safe, efficient, and satisfying swallow or by altering the assumed pathophysiology underlying the abnormal swallow. For example, if weakness or reduced endurance were posited to be the reason for swallowing signs in an individual patient, then a rehabilitative technique is one that improves strength or endurance. This approach is in contrast to a compensation approach in which impaired skill, strength, or endurance would simply

55

be accommodated by postural change, diet modification, or some other alteration in how or what the patient is eating and drinking. In addition to strength or endurance, rehabilitative techniques involve efforts to change sensory thresholds, tone, timing, or coordination. Chapter 14 contains descriptions of the rehabilitative procedures potentially useful in movement disorders. The challenges of evaluating rehabilitative treatment effects are similar to those for the compensatory methods. However, the clinician faces other challenges as well. The foremost of these is that rehabilitation usually requires more of the clinician's and patient's time than do compensatory methods, and the effects are often delayed by weeks. As but one example, it may take

6 or more weeks for strength to improve, despite nearly daily exercise.

A final challenge in executing intelligent treatments, especially rehabilitative ones, is that traditional training often ignores the principles that guide such treatments. Students are taught how to do the techniques but not how to select them or how to evaluate new techniques when they appear, often to great clinical acclaim. Therefore, the next two chapters (Chapter 10 and Chapter 11) offer brief lists of principles for both compensatory and rehabilitative approaches. Once learned, they seldom need to be reconsulted, but the rewards of reading these chapters carefully may be substantial. It may prevent use of ineffective or otherwise inappropriate methodologies.

10 Principles of Compensatory Treatments

Compensatory as used in this chapter refers to approaches that try to accommodate each person's dysphagia rather than trying to improve it. Three broad classes of activity traditionally are defined as compensatory:

1. *The first is change in posture.* The usual ones described in the treatment literature are the *head turn* and *chin tuck.* The goal of such adjustments is to put a patient in a posture that allows safer, more efficient passage of the bolus through the mouth and pharynx and into the esophagus.
2. *The second is change in the food and/or liquid preparation.* The usual changes are in food consistency— regular, mechanical, soft, pureed— and in the viscosity of the liquid using thickeners.
3. *The third is change in approach to eating.* Any number of manipulations fit here. Common sense changes are bolus size, rate of eating or drinking, and bolus order, such as when liquids and solids are alternated.

To the casual practitioner making these changes may seem simple enough, so simple that principles should not be necessary. We believe, however, that deci-

sions about compensatory approaches are (or should be) difficult. These difficult decisions may be improved if made with a few principles in mind.

PRINCIPLE 1

The classification of all swallowing treatments into rehabilitative and compensatory is based on tradition and not on data. Therefore, the classification is likely to be wrong. Consider the use of thickened liquids. It is assumed that their use is compensatory. The patient, for example, who aspirates thin liquids and is placed on thickened liquids may well be safer. It is possible he may also swallow more than if placed NPO (*nil per os* or, more commonly, nothing per oral). Does increased swallowing translate into improved swallowing? The answer to this question remains unknown, but we suspect continuing to swallow food and drink is more beneficial than remaining NPO and reducing the number of swallows completed. This may be especially true if the clinician couples an altered diet with instruction that the swallows be quicker, more complete, or in some other way more skillful.

PRINCIPLE 2

Despite principle 1, *we advocate using rehabilitative treatments before or in consort with compensatory ones as a first order of clinical business.* For example, in the case of a patient needing thickened liquids because of aspiration through an inadequate laryngeal valve, a rehabilitation program to increase laryngeal closure should be introduced if the patient has even a modest chance of understanding and completing it.

PRINCIPLE 3

Not all compensations, even if they appear effective on the videofluoroscopic swallow examination (VFSE), will keep a patient safe from the effects of aspiration. The rule is that aspirators aspirate. Additionally, as noted by Logemann and colleagues (2008), the effect of aspiration of thickened liquids remains unknown and may increase the likelihood of pulmonary complications.

PRINCIPLE 4

Compensatory techniques, especially if they involve postural adjustments, may be unacceptable to some patients. In this case, the clinician is wise to select one or more rehabilitative techniques exclusively or do nothing.

PRINCIPLE 5

If selected, the planned duration of compensatory techniques should be considered and that duration explained to the patient prior to introduction. If a compensatory technique is not rehabilitative, at least for an individual patient, and is therefore likely to be part of the patient's swallowing for a lifetime, the patient should know that. Few of us would choose to tuck our chins for years on end.

PRINCIPLE 6

Combinations of compensatory techniques or of compensatory and rehabilitative techniques are likely to have the greatest positive effect. For example, a chin tuck and head turn combined with thickened liquids and a laryngeal closing technique may constitute a total therapy for an individual.

PRINCIPLE 7

Lack of patient compliance with compensatory methods is likely to be high. Evaluating the acceptability of any suggestions about compensations and avoiding their use when a patient is clearly unresponsive may save dollars, time, and travail.

11 Principles of Rehabilitative Techniques

Rehabilitative techniques are of two basic types, depending on target. *Type one techniques* aim to change the underlying pathophysiology, principally weakness and reduced endurance. *Type two techniques* aim to increase skill. To achieve either aim, treatments must be guided by one or more of a limited number of principles. These principles derive from what is known about how to influence *plasticity*, or a person's ability to change with experience. We identify three kinds of plasticity: *muscle*, *behavioral*, and *neural*. This chapter contains a description of principles that guide efforts to influence one or more of these three kinds of plasticity. We felt compelled to review them because treatments independent of such principles are likely to be useless at best and dangerous at worst. All methods do not conform to all principles, nor should they. Indeed, methods may seem to fit some and violate others. In this latter incidence, it is up to the clinician to make choices about how to proceed. Please refer to Chapter 14 for more details on the rehabilitative methods discussed below.

MUSCLE PLASTICITY

Muscle plasticity as used in this volume, refers to *chemical, cellular, and muscle fiber changes secondary to appropriate training to increase strength and endurance*. Two main principles govern treatment to improve strength or endurance.

The first principle is *specificity*. In its simplest form, specificity refers to the phenomenon that persons improve the specific behaviors they practice. The implication for swallowing is that *treatment targets should ideally include components of the behavior to be improved, swallowing in this case*. According to this criterion, tongue protrusion and lateralization against the resistance of a tongue blade fail to meet the specificity principle, as swallowing does not require these two movements. The hard swallow, on the other hand, does meet the criterion. Lee Silverman Voice Therapy (LSVT) approximates it in at least one way: it requires, as does swallowing, laryngeal adduction. Tongue strengthening using the Iowa Oral Performance Instrument (IOPI) (Robin, Goel, Somodi, & Luschei, 1992; Robin, Somodi, & Luschei, 1991) also satisfies this criterion, as strengthening of tongue tip and tongue back elevation is the goal. Using a method that fails to meet the specificity principle is not necessarily to be avoided. On the other hand, influence of methods that violate the principle may be slow to work and their effects minimal or even nonexistent. Clinicians need to decide if they can risk these outcomes with methods failing to meet the specificity criterion. In favor of many such methods, however, is that they may conform to another principle, that of overload.

The second principle, *overload*, guides all procedures whose aim is strengthening or increasing endurance. Overload means *the treatment requires more strength or endurance than is necessary for the normal performance of that task*. Simply swallowing, unless it is against resistance or in some other way made more difficult, fails to meet the overload principle. Therefore, the classic notion that swallowing is the best treatment for swallowing needs to be critically evaluated. On the other hand, the Masako maneuver, during which the person swallows with his tongue protruded, conforms to the principle because successfully swallowing in this manner is very difficult. Similarly, expiratory muscle strength training (EMST) meets this criterion by requiring the person to exhale against systematically increasing resistance.

Other principles are assumed within the overload principle. Selected ones of these are worth reviewing, despite our near total ignorance about how they apply in swallowing rehabilitation.

One of these concerns is the *amount of resistance* to be added to the performance for strength to increase. The guideline borrowed from the physical training literature is that training should occur at 60–75% of maximum strength (Powers & Howley, 2003). Most of the traditional strength training procedures, such as using tongue blades to resist tongue protrusion as one example, are seldom applied in light of this principle. Newer methods, such as respiratory muscle strength training or tongue strengthening with the IOPI, however, can be. And

it may even be that strengthening with a tongue blade can be made to meet this criterion at least roughly, and roughly may be sufficient (Lazarus, Logemann, Huang, & Rademaker, 2003).

A second principle is *intensity*. At a minimum, rehabilitative treatments, especially those to improve strength or endurance, should be conducted for 6 weeks. Longer is almost always better. Similarly, a minimum number of sessions per week is three, and six is preferable, though most need not be completed in the clinic. Finally, the number of repetitions per day has never been established in the swallowing literature, but our rule of thumb is a minimum of 25 per day for strengthening and 100 per day (at a lower load) for endurance. Clearly, these are rigorous requirements and much beyond the clinician's time or third-party payer resources. Hence the absolute necessity of a home therapy program accompanied by a diary, so that each patient can record the number of repetitions per day, number of days per week, and number of weeks over which treatment is extended. Patients must of course return to the clinic regularly, so that gains can be measured and new targets, such as amount of resistance, established.

A third is the *necessity for continuing exercise* if maintenance is to be established. Strength and endurance decline when training stops. Therefore, maintenance programs are a necessity. The intensity of these can be reduced and clinical follow-up is often unnecessary. This principle can be discouraging for patients. Many are not compliant with this notion and some will refuse to enter into a treatment once they know the obligation. It is a form of clinical dishonesty, however, to initiate certain programs without mentioning the maintenance principle.

Reminding patients of their experiences in the gym may make the principle clear, even though it may remain unacceptable.

BEHAVIORAL PLASTICITY

Behavioral plasticity refers to *the body's ability to change performance under the influence of experience*. The critical performance in this text is improved swallowing, and the experience is treatment. One way to think about behavioral plasticity is in relation to skill. The conceptual payoff for viewing improved swallowing as improved skill is that the principles governing skill learning are beginning to be discovered and can be applied to swallowing therapy. While the viability of these principles is still to be demonstrated in dysphagia, it seems prudent to introduce them here, because they make good therapeutic sense and help clinicians organize how they are applying any one of several popular treatments.

Principle 1 is that the *number and spacing of repetitions* of the target behavior seems to be important. It is probably safe to say that 25 repetitions a day, 6 days per week for 6 weeks, is an absolute minimum for any kind of training. We usually recommend more repetitions, often twice as many. The spacing of treatments, that is, whether the treatment should be massed with multiple repetitions completed each day several days in a row or distributed with fewer sessions per day over a longer period, for example, has never been addressed in the swallowing treatment literature. Therefore, a simple rule can be a guide. Massed practice may make for quick acquisition but submaximal retention.

Spaced practice may slow acquisition but make for improved retention at the end of treatment. Clinicians need to decide what they want at each stage of treatment for each patient. When first beginning with a patient, especially one with significant difficulty, quick acquisition may be the best goal. More widely distributed practice as the patient gains competence also makes sense.

Principle 2 is that *knowledge of results* (KR) and *knowledge of performance* (KP) are important in skill learning and may differentially affect swallowing training as well. KR is merely providing information about whether a response was adequate or inadequate. Clinicians use it all the time when they encourage patients with "Nice job," "Good," "Not quite," and the like. KR includes nothing about the nature of the performance physiologically. In contrast, KP provides more specific information about the quality of the movement produced, such as feedback about how a behavior like a swallow in response to the clinician's directions has been performed. The feedback can be verbal (e.g., "You failed to hold your larynx high in your neck for the full 2 seconds.") or physiologic ("This [electromyographic trace] shows that the amount of muscle force from the muscles under your chin failed to meet our goal."). KP is especially useful for physiologic performance such as swallowing, where most movements are invisible and must be inferred from observations such as wet voice or throat clearing. KP may also have a more robust influence on retention than does KR. Little information is available about the differential effects of these two forms of feedback on swallowing, with the exception of the relative effect of surface electromyography (sEMG) to deliver KP in training the

Mendelsohn maneuver as compared to traditional feedback, which is either verbal KP or more likely simple KR. It may well turn out that KP, either verbal or in the form of a physiologic feedback such as sEMG, is preferable, especially for the most severe cases of dysphagia.

Principle 3 is that the *timing of feedback will influence acquisition and retention of trained responses*. For example, it is known that timing of feedback influences normal skill acquisition, with delayed and summary feedback being associated with greater retention than immediate feedback after every trial. By delaying feedback, the patient is given the opportunity for self-evaluation, an advantage that also resides with summary feedback, in which two or more responses are elicited before the clinician provides feedback. Self-evaluation may well make improved performance easier to do outside the clinic. Unfortunately, most clinicians have never been taught about the importance of timing and so usually provide immediate feedback, most often in the form of KR, after each response. It can be argued that such behavior actually threatens the carryover of responses acquired in the clinic to the world outside it. It is important to note, however, that no data on this variable are available in swallowing. Clinicians are left to follow their best clinical hunches.

NEURAL PLASTICITY

Behavior change is impossible without neural change. Not surprisingly, therefore, the principles of *neural plasticity* overlap with those of behavioral plasticity. We review them below, however, because there are some differences. We also review them

because as treatments and our understanding of their effects get more sophisticated, we predict the profession will need to attend to both forms of plasticity. It is already being posited that behavioral plasticity precedes the form of neural plasticity associated with relative permanence of a treatment gain. The implication is that training must continue beyond the time that behavioral criteria, such as reaching an 80% success rate during each of three consecutive sessions, would lead us to believe. Neural plasticity is the "*adaptive capacity of the central nervous system*" (Kleim & Jones, 2008, p. S225).

The principles of neural plasticity have been outlined by Kleim and Jones (2008), and this discussion is nearly totally dependent on their original discussion. Table 11–1 contains the principles and a brief discussion of each.

Principle 1: Use It or Lose It

This is nearly a cliché, but a useful one, especially in dysphagia, where some clinicians believe that nonoral nutrition is always safe nutrition. Inherent in this principle is that nervous system networks are precious real estate and if the behavior they are used to support is no longer performed or is performed with drastically decreased frequency, that neural tissue will be usurped by some other behavior. Therefore, clinicians must consider the fate of the neural structures serving swallowing when they are part of a tube-feeding decision. This is not to say that nonoral nutrition is ill-advised. It is to say that such a decision may have nervous system consequences. These include the diversion of neural substrate to other behaviors and perhaps the need to begin swallow rehabilitation immediately.

Table 11–1. Principles of neural plasticity as developed by Kleim and Jones (2008)	
Principle	*Description*
1. Use It or Lose It	Failure to drive specific brain functions can lead to functional degradation.
2. Use It and Improve It	Training that drives a specific brain function can lead to an enhancement of that function.
3. Specificity Matters	The nature of the training experience dictates the nature of the plasticity.
4. Repetition Matters	Induction of plasticity requires sufficient repetition.
5. Intensity Matters	Induction of plasticity requires sufficient training intensity.
6. Time Matters	Different forms of plasticity occur at different times during training.
7. Salience Matters	The training experience must be sufficiently salient to induce plasticity.
8. Age Matters	Training-induced plasticity occurs more readily in younger brains.
9. Transference	Plasticity in response to one training experience can enhance the acquisition of similar behaviors.
10. Interference	Plasticity in response to one experience can interfere with the acquisition of other behaviors.

Note. From "Principles of Experience-Dependent Neural Plasticity: Implications for Rehabilitation after Brain Damage," by J. A. Kleim and T. A. Jones, *Journal of Speech, Language, and Hearing Research*, *51*(1), p. S227. Copyright 2008 by American Speech-Language-Hearing Association. All rights reserved. Reprinted with permission.

Principle 2: Use It and Improve It

This can be the rallying cry of rehabilitationists. Nervous system support of improved function occurs in response to intelligent treatment. No longer is the adult nervous system seen as immutable. It changes with practice and those changes support improved performance, even in those with neurological disease. One important issue in dysphagia management is the degree to which compensatory activities such as swallowing with a chin tuck and head turn have the same positive effect on neural structures as do intensive rehabilitation techniques to improve swallowing function. Until the issue is resolved, we recommend aggressive treatment for all patients who want and can cooperate with it.

Principle 3: Specificity Matters

Simply put, this principle says that a person gets better at doing what he is trained to do. Other kinds of performance are unlikely to improve unless they are similar to the treated response. Therefore, training swallowing and swallowing-related movements are better targets of treatment than movements only casually or unrelated to those required for swallowing.

Principle 4: Repetition Matters

Once is not enough. This principle is the same as that included in the preceding behavioral plasticity section.

Principle 5: Intensity Matters

This is true in driving neural plasticity, just as it is in driving behavioral plasticity. At issue, however, is whether the intensity that brings acquisition of a behavioral response as usually defined is accompanied by sufficient neural plasticity to support the behavior maximally after treatment has ended. The answer must await further research.

Principle 6: Time Matters

This principle has multiple meanings. At what point treatment is introduced after onset of a condition such as dysphagia also matters, but rehabilitationists are ignorant of the subtleties. It continues to be common practice to assume that early intervention is preferable to later intervention. Probably that is true. However, the data on the possible neurotoxic effects of exercise in rats following experimentally induced stroke is sobering (Bland et al., 1998; Kozlowski, James, & Schallert, 1996), though this has not been found in rodent models of Parkinson's disease (Sasco, Paffenbarger, Gendre, & Wing, 1992).

Principle 7: Salience Matters

Nervous system response is likely to be greater to meaningful rather than meaningless or less meaningful tasks. Therefore, swallowing as part of eating is likely to be more powerful than swallowing alone. Saliva swallowing is likely to be more therapeutic than merely swallowing upon command. Whole swallows are likely to be more therapeutic than portions of swallowing movements. This principle, of course, must be evaluated within the context of what is safe.

Principle 8: Age Matters

It is true that younger nervous systems are more plastic than older ones, but age should never influence the decision to treat, as change is possible regardless of age. It just may be easier to change the young brain in comparison to the older brain.

Principle 9: Transference

Another way of designating this principle is the concept of generalization. Treatment of one behavior may generalize to similar behaviors. Hence, increased skill in safely swallowing one bolus type or viscosity may transfer to improved skill with another. Generalization has limits, of course, and the more unlike two behaviors are, the less likely it is that transference will occur.

Principle 10: Interference

In other words, changes in one system may inhibit changes in another. To our knowledge, neural interference has never been demonstrated in dysphagia; however, it is not difficult to imagine. Some versions of hard swallow, as when the patient is asked to force his tongue against the roof of the mouth as hard as possible before executing a swallow, is disruptive of the swallow for some persons. Presumably the disruption occurs because a static posture (pressing the tongue against the palate) is imposed on what is an exquisitely complex action. This interference is easy to see behaviorally. The influence on neural networks can only be imagined.

SUMMARY

This short chapter has highlighted a series of principles applicable to dyspha-gia treatment. They were not drawn from the dysphagia treatment literature because that literature remains limited. Indeed, about the only principle discoverable in that literature is that treatment should be directed at the presumed abnormal physiology underlying the signs of abnormal swallowing. That principle is a useful one, but it is insufficient. It may direct one generally to a method but be mute on how the method is to be applied. The additional guidelines contained in this chapter are meant to provide a basis for clinicians as they select traditional methods or try to decide whether or not to adopt new or recently popular treatments and, if so, how to do them for maximum effect.

12 General Treatment Considerations

Treatment decisions are not guided solely by the principles outlined in the previous chapters. Although movement disorders differ one from another, certain features of the disorders and their medical, surgical, and behavioral management generate general treatment considerations. Like the principles, these more general considerations influence treatment planning and execution more or less regardless of medical diagnosis. Hence, they are included in a separate chapter to avoid needless redundancy in the specific disorder chapters.

TEAM PLANNING

Movement disorders, especially in major medical centers, are managed by interdisciplinary teams of neurologists, neurosurgeons, neuropsychologists, physical and occupational therapists, nurses, and speech-language pathologists. Therefore, decisions about swallowing therapy can be made only in light of what the entire team is planning. Once a clinician has seen and examined a patient to determine if a behavioral treatment may be necessary, we recommend the following steps.

Ask questions of the patient and caregiver to determine the medical/surgical treatment plan, its timeline, and what their expectations of that treatment are.

Some patients may not know this information, but their caregivers may. Additionally, this information is likely to be in the medical record. In some cases, professional consultation will be required to obtain this information.

Recognize that if medications are being adjusted or surgery planned, then waiting (except in extreme cases of dysphagia) until maximum treatment effects have been achieved may be advisable. Medications and surgery can have variable effects on swallowing function in Parkinson's disease (PD) and other movement disorders. Both can make (or seem to make) swallowing better, worse, or leave it unaffected. The effect for an individual patient should be established with maximum possible confidence during history and observation and evaluation before treatment is planned.

Once the effect is established, the patient, family, and clinician need to decide if behavioral treatment is also justified. The answer is usually "Yes" when medications or surgery have made swallowing worse or when swallowing is functionally impaired and unimproved by medications or surgery. The answer may be "Yes" or "No" when medical treatment or surgery improves swallowing, depending on the amount of improvement. For those conditions where medical and surgical treatments are unavailable or inappropriate and in which swallowing is functionally impaired, the answer is "Yes" if the swallowing deficit is influencing eating adequacy, safety, or pleasure.

"Yes" to behavioral treatment may be appropriate under one other condition as well. It may be that exercise as is required by most behavioral treatments has a *neuroprotective effect.* As Smith and Zigmond (2003) say, data "raise the possibility that exercise will protect against a variety of neurodegenerative conditions" (p. 31). This possibility is being evaluated in a variety of laboratories. In the interim, professionals such as Farley and colleagues (in press) are advocating the early initiation of exercise programs for those diagnosed with PD. If one believes in the potential neuroprotective effect of exercise, then treatment early in a disease's course rather than late should be considered.

A COMBINATION OF TECHNIQUES

Dysphagia treatment in the movement disorders is *often a combination of compensatory and rehabilitative techniques.* Three conditions prompt this dual approach.

Compensatory approaches may allow the person to continue eating while rehabilitative approaches are building a physiologic base for more normal, safe, or enjoyable nutrition. For example, while aspiration is being treated with laryngeal closure rehabilitation techniques, thickened liquids or use of a chin tuck may be critical to swallowing adequacy and safety in the interim. A rehabilitative technique may be only partially helpful, and safety and adequacy of nutrition may require a simultaneous set of compensatory adjustments. In some cases, rehabilitation may have limited effects and compensations will be the only way of helping the person to continue eating successfully.

MOVEMENT DISORDERS ARE PROGRESSIVE

Most movement disorders are progressive, implying that rehabilitative techniques will need to occur over a long time, be introduced multiple times in a disease's course, or be combined with compensatory approaches as outlined above. Furthermore, disease progression will often require that the exact methodology and expectations of treatment need constant readjustment. For example, modest improvement in swallowing adequacy or even slowing decline may be respectable outcomes in the degenerative movement disorders.

REEVALUATION

Frequent reevaluation is also critical. Most of these disorders change over time and a dysphagia may go from being of little significance to having a substantial impact on safety, adequacy, or pleasure of eating and drinking in a short time. Medical and surgical treatments may affect the swallow in a positive way for a period, only to lose that affect. Behavioral treatment may have greater effects at some periods in a disease's course than others, and a behavioral treatment may even have positive effects during some portions of a typical day and no affect at other times. All these patterns of variability prompt systematic reevaluation.

STOPPING TREATMENT

Knowing when or if to stop rehabilitative treatment can be difficult in most movement disorders because of their usual progressive nature. One reasonably obvious sign that treatment is having no effect is continued decline despite treatment, although it might occasionally be argued that the decline would have been steeper had treatment not been offered. A short period of treatment withdrawal may provide evidence in support of this notion. Improvement and even stability over some period of time (during which other untreated functions may show obvious decline) are evidence of a treatment effect. In those cases, rehabilitative efforts can continue, assuming patient willingness and ability to continue.

DEMENTIA

Compensations can have relatively permanent effects, although they may have to be simplified and responsibility for compliance transferred to caregivers for those with severe illness or for whom cognitive decline is part of the symptomatology.

Dementia is frequently present in the profile of those with movement disorders, especially later in the course of those who have progressive disease. Dementia sets the upper limit on what can be expected from rehabilitative methods and, if severe enough, dictates that the

approaches be compensatory only and controlled by a caregiver.

Therefore, measuring cognitive integrity is critical as a basis for prognosis and treatment planning. Depending on the facility, cognitive assessments may be conducted by neuropsychology, speech-language pathology, or both. It needs to be extensive enough to provide experienced clinicians with a hypothesis about the patient's ability to cooperate and learn. Some clinicians will prefer to try to teach a methodology and conclude such teaching is impossible only if the patient fails to learn or to generalize. This latter approach has much to recommend it.

TUBE FEEDING

Specific guidelines for recommending nonoral nutrition such as a percutaneous endoscopic gastrostomy (PEG) have never been established for patients with movement disorders. Clinicians tempted to suggest this alternative would do well to remember the following:

1. Tube feeding does not prevent aspiration but only influences what is aspirated.
2. Once nonoral nutrition has been established, tube feeding can be difficult to discontinue.
3. Rehabilitative efforts need not cease after a tube is placed and the presence of a PEG, for example, does not preclude attempts at rehabilitation.
4. Some patients can continue to take some foods and liquids by mouth in what might be called "recreational eating."
5. A tube is often seen as evidence that the end is in sight. Therefore, serious

discussions about the possibility of its contributing to a stabilization of nutrition and even improved functioning and quality of life are important.

IMPAIRED JUDGMENT

Patients with movement disorders, notably some with PD, seem to have special difficulty with perception of magnitude. The classic examples are drawn from vocal loudness experiments that inconsistently demonstrate an inability to correctly judge speech intensity. No simple clinical tool is available to evaluate such perceptual competence, but the clinician can often determine competence with simple clinical procedures requiring self-judgment.

The inability to make judgments is a profound influence on treatment because ability to judge adequacy is a key to retention of lessons learned in the clinic. Without the ability to make adequate judgments, a patient is at the mercy of external (usually clinician) input. Such dependence may be appropriate in treatment's early days, but retention of clinical gains after treatment is done depends on self-evaluation. Thus, even informal attempts to evaluate a patient's ability to respond to internally generated cues can help determine prognosis and shape treatment. Improved self-monitoring can be taught in many instances.

COMORBIDITY

Multiple complications or comorbidities are the norm in patients with movement disorders. Therefore, the swallowing clinician needs to be mindful of:

1. The need to recognize the interaction of dysphagia with these other conditions and their treatment.
2. The need to have patients rank the impact of their various conditions. If swallowing is ranked third or fourth, for example, treatment may be deferred until other conditions are managed or until its severity elevates it in the list.

OTHER CONSIDERATIONS

Referral for behavioral treatment of all symptoms, including dysphagia, in individuals with movement disorders is often deferred until medical and surgical treatments have failed. This pattern creates a significant challenge for the clinician. By the time patients are referred, their symptoms are often severe and they are resigned to them. This is not to say that prognosis is inevitably poor. It is to say that treatment may be more challenging than it is with early referral, in other nonprogressive conditions, or in those where medical/surgical treatments are less available or promising.

Sleep disturbance is not unique to movement disorders, but when it is present, prognosis for enduring treatment effects will be negatively influenced. Sleep is critical to learning, and treatment's lessons are likely to be harder to retain if sleep is disturbed. Appropriate management of sleep disturbance to the degree possible is important to all other treatments.

Encourage support group attendance, as this can provide a vital form of environmental enrichment in the form of shared stories, experiences, and insights.

Encourage general exercise, which for some may involve nothing more than being up for more hours than are spent sleeping or on the couch or recliner. Our view is that prognosis is generally better for those patients who are physically active, whether this is informal exercise or involvement in physical therapy.

Encourage socialization. Like a support group, traditional socialization can provide critical environmental enrich-ment and may foster greater receptivity to treatment. It may even be associated with better learning and retention.

By including these general principles separately, we hoped to avoid needless repetition in the specific disease chapters. The danger is, of course, that this chapter may be ignored. If so, the treatments based only on the content in the disease chapters will be incomplete.

13 Compensatory Techniques

Compensatory techniques are of three types: *postural adjustments*, *alterations in food and liquid preparation*, and *alterations in eating*. The reader is urged to examine the preceding chapters on principles, because some—such as the need for systematic reevaluation—need to be considered in all instances, but to have included those procedures in this chapter would have led to unsatisfactory redundancy.

POSTURAL ADJUSTMENTS

Posture is usually adjusted to improve bolus flow, but in movement disorders, certain adjustments may also improve transfer of the bolus to the mouth.

Chin Tuck

The chin tuck, in which the patient lowers his head toward or until it touches the chest, threatens to become the universal approach to compensation. "Threatens" is used because the method is being adopted *uncritically* as the first suggestion in the presence of dysphagia from a variety of different causes and with different signs and underlying pathophysi-

ology. It is important to remember that a chin tuck can actually make dysphagia worse in some patients, especially those who aspirate material from the pyriform sinuses or who have difficulty retaining a bolus in the mouth without allowing it to leak between the lips.

Description of the Method

The method seems, on the surface, to be simple. The patient typically takes or is provided with a bolus and then executes a chin tuck prior to swallowing. Urging the patient toward the best extent of tuck and reinforcing the same amount of tuck and the appropriate timing prior to the swallow constitute the usual additional features for a successful performance.

Modifications

Modifications are few in number. Remarkably, the most frequent modification seems to be the amount of tuck. Even when a problem of the cervical spine does not limit the tuck, the amount encouraged by different clinicians may well differ. In our view, the amount of tuck should be established, wherever possible, during videofluoroscopic swallow examination (VFSE). Generally, the closer the chin is to the chest, the better.

An exception is when a person has limited ability to retain the bolus in the mouth. Too extreme a tuck in that case may result in the bolus leaking from the mouth. A quick tuck like that taken by non-dysphagic swallowers, often when taking pills, may be a better postural adjustment than methodically tucking the chin, holding the posture, and then swallowing.

Another modification may be the frequency of tucking. Most people, in our experience, find it difficult to tuck their chins with every swallow. Because most people do not have dysphagia so severely that every swallow of every bolus is threatening to their safety, the best approach may be to use the tuck only during the swallowing of those boluses that represent the greatest challenge.

Frequency and Duration

If this maneuver makes the swallow safer, more efficient, or more satisfying and if rehabilitation is not possible, is ongoing, or has been unsuccessful, the frequency and duration decisions are relatively simple. The maneuver needs to be employed on all hard to swallow boluses until rehabilitation makes the posture unnecessary, until the swallow improves because of time or medical/surgical treatment, or until the patient tires of the inconvenience.

Candidacy

In our experience the best candidates are those who:

1. Need to eat while they are being rehabilitated and who have demonstrated clearly superior swallowing in this posture.
2. Penetrate or aspirate before or during the swallow because of a delay in swallow initiation or poor airway closure.
3. Have reduced tongue base retraction at swallow initiation.

Those who aspirate material from the pyriform sinuses before, during, or after the swallow may not benefit and may indeed be made worse.

Effects

The chin tuck can:

1. Shorten and narrow the pharynx, thereby helping to protect the larynx.
2. Improve the force of suprahyoid musculature contraction because of muscle shortening.
3. Increase laryngeal closure.

Potentially the result of all these changes is to reduce the amount of pharyngeal residue and the number or severity of penetration and aspiration events after the swallow.

The Evidence

A recent systematic review assessed the effect data of the chin tuck in healthy individuals (Ashford et al., submitted). This review examined studies of healthy subjects from Bulow, Olsson, and Ekberg (1999), Castell and colleagues (1993), and Welch and colleagues (1993). In comparison to normal swallows, the chin tuck resulted in increased "pharyngeal contraction pressure, the duration of pharyngeal contraction pressure, [and] larynx to hyoid bone distance" (Ashford et al., submitted). The effects of the chin tuck have also been studied in individuals with dysphagia (Bulow, Olsson, & Ekberg, 2001,

2002; Ertekin et al., 2001; Rasley et al., 1993). For example, Ertekin and colleagues (2001) measured the effect of chin tuck, chin elevation, and left and right head turn electromyographically in 51 patients with neurogenic dysphagia. Forty-two had bilateral as opposed to unilateral oropharyngeal weakness. Of the 42 with bilateral involvement, 5 had Parkinson's disease (PD) and an additional 7 had various other movement disorders. Fifty percent of the bilateral patients could safely take larger boluses of water in the chin tuck position. Specific effects for those with movement disorders are not reported. The *chin up* position, it is worth noting, did not have therapeutic effects. Data from Bulow and colleagues (2001, 2002) are perhaps less encouraging. They studied the effect of various postures and maneuvers for dysphagia, including the chin tuck, on pharyngeal pressure. At the level of the inferior pharyngeal constrictor, the peak or duration of pharyngeal pressure in a small number of patients with dysphagia secondary to stroke or head and neck cancer was not altered. It is important to remember that the best test of the method's effect is how each individual patient responds.

Head Turn (Rotation)

Description of Method

In its simplest form, the patient is instructed to turn his head either to the right or left side ("Look over your right (or left) shoulder.") prior to swallowing. Logemann and colleagues (1989) recommend 90° of rotation. Once the swallow is complete, the head is returned to the forward position.

Modifications

Typically, the side of the turn is determined by the side of greatest weakness or other involvement in those patients with a substantial asymmetry. Systematically evaluating the effect of turning the head first to one side and then the other is good diagnostic policy. Often it is impossible to predict which turn will have the best effect without comparing them carefully. Combining the head turn with the chin tuck may be a maximally effective procedure in some instances. Amount of head turn may also influence the effect.

Frequency and Duration

This is the same as with the chin tuck. Patients usually object to doing it on every swallow, so tailoring when possible the type of bolus to the need for the maneuver can help with compliance. Frequent follow-up is mandatory to make sure the posture is still necessary.

Candidacy

Candidacy is determined by the following:

1. Swallowing asymmetry on the anterior-posterior (A-P) view
2. Asymmetry accompanied by large postswallow residuals anywhere in the laryngopharynx or pyriform sinuses
3. Asymmetry accompanied by poor airway protection with penetration or aspiration before, during, or after the swallow
4. Rehabilitation that is impossible or anticipated to occur with unacceptable slowness

Effects

Effects have not been established in any of the movement disorders, although some studies (Rasley et al., 1993) have used mixed neurologic etiologies. The bolus may be directed to the better side of the swallowing tube, with decreased pressure within the upper esophageal sphincter (UES) and increased width of UES opening, thereby reducing residual after the swallow and perhaps reducing risk of aspiration after the swallow.

The Evidence

A recent systematic review assessed the effect data of the head turn in healthy individuals (Ashford et al., submitted). Studies by Logemann et al. (1989) and Ohame and colleagues (1998) found that in nondysphagic subjects, the head turn "resulted in increased pharyngeal contraction pressure at the level of the valleculae and pyriform sinuses on side of rotation, decreased UES resting pressure on the side opposite rotation, increased duration from peak pharyngeal pressure . . . to the end of UES relaxation, and increased UES anterior-posterior opening diameter" (Ashford et al., submitted). Rasley et al. (1993) studied the head turn along with other postural adjustments in a mix of 165 patients with neurologic diagnoses, presumably some with movement disorders. Postural modifications, including rotation, resulted in decreased occurrence of aspiration. Overall, the evidence for the effect of this treatment is limited and it should be applied with caution. Probably the least therapeutic effect will be seen in those with bilateral involvement, and unfortunately bilateral involvement is present in the majority of movement disorders, especially as the disease progresses and treatment is most necessary.

Head and Body Stabilization

Description of Methods

Patients with a variety of movement disorders may get some benefit from efforts to stabilize the head or body. The most extreme example is the *geste antagoniste* or sensory trick, variable from patient to patient, that is associated with at least a temporary normalization of dystonic posturing. We have seen a patient whose dystonia resolved when he held his cell phone to his ear, whether or not it was turned on, as but one dramatic example. Holding a toothpick between the teeth has also been described multiple times as a sensory trick for oromandibular dystonia (see Chapter 18 for more on dystonia). Clinicians seldom have to discover these, as patients often arrive knowing what, if anything, reduces their movements. Usually less dramatic are the postural adjustments for other conditions. The following can be tried:

1. Resting the chin on the hand while chewing and swallowing
2. Resting the head against a high-back chair or even against the wall while chewing and swallowing
2. Side lying, which has been described in the head and neck cancer literature and may be useful in movement disorders

Modifications

Any other posture that stabilizes or otherwise reduces abnormal movements in the head, its various parts, or the body may be tried in accompaniment to getting food to the mouth, preparing it for the swallow, and swallowing.

Frequency and Duration

The same rules apply as to the other postural adjustments. This approach is best used selectively and its effects evaluated systematically.

Candidacy

Candidates include anyone whose disrupted swallow is better with the postural adjustment and those whose medical team decides they will not suffer a worsening of the movement with protracted postural adjustment.

Effects

As will be shown, the data are very limited. However, it can be posited that effects may include getting food to the mouth, chewing or otherwise forming it efficiently, and improved movement of the bolus posteriorly in the mouth and through the pharynx into the esophagus. These results may occur because the posture leads to a reduction in the movement abnormality. Swallowing may also improve because the patient is free to concentrate more on swallowing than is possible when trying to control the movement abnormality volitionally, with subsequent improvement in getting food or drink to the mouth, preparing it for swallowing, and swallowing.

The Evidence

To our knowledge, no evidence exists. Therefore, each patient must become an experiment of one.

MODIFICATION OF SOLIDS AND LIQUIDS

Changing food preparation (pureeing it, for example) and altering the viscosity of liquids are probably the most frequent procedures clinicians employ in response to dysphagia from any cause, including movement disorders.

Description of the Methods

Diet changes are usually made in the interest of patient safety. Seldom do they accomplish the goals of efficiency or satisfaction, although efficiency may be more frequently improved than is pleasure. The methods are relatively straightforward on the surface, but it is important for clinicians to recognize that most diet changes are made based on intuition. A problem is that the validity of those changes is seldom established. In other words, a clinician makes an educated guess about the proper diet using, most frequently, results from the VFSE and clinical experience. However, the VFSE is seldom sufficient to the task of diet planning. At very least, the results must be combined with as many other pieces of information as possible. The method of reaching diet change decisions in what is admittedly an ideal situation is outlined below.

A chart review and history can establish with a fair degree of confidence whether the patient will accept an altered diet if one is recommended. Recall that patients have control over decisions affecting their health care. The review and history will also establish the individual patient's risk of illness from aspiration if it occurs.

A thorough clinical swallow examination (CSE), including eating trials with a variety of solid and liquid boluses, will provide some information about real-world swallowing and its dangers, as well as insight into approaches that might make eating safer, more efficient, or more pleasurable.

A VFSE or videoendoscopic swallow examination can establish the integrity of swallowing physiology, at least for the boluses and conditions of the test. It can also identify penetration and aspiration of test materials. Unfortunately, it cannot tell the clinician whether aspiration or penetration occurs on those or any other material at any other time.

When all this information is assembled and integrated, the clinician, in concert with the patient, family, and other members of the health care team, will be able to decide about a recommendation for maintaining or modifying solids and liquids.

According to the National Dysphagia Diet (NDD) guidelines from the National Dysphagia Diet Task Force (2002), the following choices for standardized food consistencies are:

1. NDD Level I: Dysphagia—pureed, very little chewing required
2. NDD Level 2: Dysphagia—mechanically altered, semisolid foods requiring some chewing
3. NDD Level 3: Dysphagia—advanced, soft foods that require more chewing
4. Regular: All foods allowed

According to guidelines from the National Dysphagia Diet Task Force (2002), the following choices for standardized liquid viscosities are:

1. Thin: viscosity of 1 to 50 centiPoise (cP)

2. Nectar-like: viscosity of 51 to 350 cP
3. Honey-like: viscosity of 351 to 1750 cP
4. Spoon-thick: viscosity of greater than 1750 cP

Systematic follow-up is important to determine if any modified diet can be liberalized or if any diet choice needs to be altered. A trial to determine the appropriateness of a liberalized diet when a restricted one has been recommended is also appropriate.

Modifications

Because the subtle modifications in this approach are so numerous, this section could be expanded substantially. However, only what seem to us to be major modifications are included below:

1. Medications may influence swallowing, so diet modification in movement disorders responsive to treatment should be evaluated in relation to medication schedule.
2. Thicker is not always better, as was demonstrated by Logemann and colleagues (2008) in a study that included PD patients with and without dementia.
3. Water can be considered even when all other liquids are being thickened.
4. Presumed safety of any viscosity change will need to be considered against the background of the challenge to compliance such changes may create. Patients often reject pureed foods and thickened liquids. The resulting malnutrition or dehydration is an assault against health as surely as is aspiration pneumonia.
5. The most normal, attractive diet possible should always be the goal.

Frequency and Duration

Generally, modified diets are necessary at all meals. The exception may be if a particular patient has very good times during which a more normal diet might be appropriate. In addition, as noted above, periodic reevaluation to see if diet can be "advanced" is appropriate.

Candidacy

Different clinicians have different criteria for candidacy given their values, training, and institutional patterns of practice. Candidacy generally can include:

1. Patient willingness to comply.
2. History of pulmonary complications because of documented or strongly suspected prandial aspiration.
3. History of malnutrition and/or dehydration.
4. Vulnerability to illness from aspiration (see Chapter 4).
5. Best possible evidence that safety will be improved by diet modification. This evidence is not easily obtained unless one does a trial of more than one diet. This difficulty is not trivial. It may be that thick liquids actually increase fatigue over time and puree may lack sufficient stimulus value to stimulate a consistently better swallow than a food preparation that requires chewing and has edges and increased structure.

Effects

The best possible effect is that altered diets reduce potentially harmful aspiration while preserving the patient's ability to eat and drink. These effects are not guaranteed.

The Evidence

Though evidence is limited, anti-PD medications appear to have a variable effect on swallowing, including a worsening (Lim, Leow, Huckabee, Frampton, & Anderson, 2008). Recent evidence also suggests that half of PD patients may not experience reduced aspiration with a chin tuck (on thin liquids) or either nectar- or honey-thick liquids. However, honey-thick liquids may more likely reduce aspiration than nectar-thick, as demonstrated in a large randomized study of men and women with PD, with and without dementia (Logemann et al., 2008). Otherwise, evidence of food and liquid alterations is in short supply.

ALTERATIONS IN EATING AND DRINKING

Sometimes safety can be preserved along with efficiency and pleasure by changing the way people eat. This section offers some suggestions.

Description of the Methods

Changing the approach to eating can sometimes be as effective as changing what is eaten. One or more of the following can be tried.

1. Smaller boluses
2. Smaller or larger sips of liquid
3. Multiple, sequential swallows rather than individual swallows
4. Sucking liquids from a straw, with or without the chin tuck or head turn
5. Use of special eating utensils such as weighted spoons to help with tremor control

6. Multiple, small meals rather than the traditional three square meals per day
7. Alternating sips and bites
8. Throat clearing after each bite or sip or after a limited number, depending on whether client feels something is stuck or in airway
9. Changing the temperature of food or drink by making it hotter, colder, or more neutral
10. Dropping troublesome food or drink from the diet
11. Eating at special times when medications are having maximum effect or when fatigue is least
12. Adding extra or fewer spices, depending on the effect
13. Locating each bolus in the "best" part of the mouth, either forward or more toward the rear and either left or right

Modifications

These are left to individual clinician creativity.

Candidacy

Candidates are those willing to make changes and for whom the changes seem to have a positive effect on swallowing (e.g., reduction in penetration or aspiration events) or on the effort associated with eating and drinking.

Effects

These changes may make eating safer, more efficient, or more pleasurable.

The Evidence

There is none we know of. Each patient will need to be evaluated and the hard decisions made.

14 Rehabilitation Techniques

This chapter summarizes rehabilitative techniques. Those rehabilitation techniques requiring special instrumentation or special certification are briefly described and references included so the interested reader can consult primary sources. Those that require clinician knowledge and a minimum of instrumentation are described more completely. Admittedly, a bit of magic goes into the division of rehabilitative and compensatory. Traditionally, and in this volume, changes in food texture or fluid viscosity are not included as rehabilitation techniques. However, there is no evidence at all that some such changes are devoid of rehabilitative function. Indeed, we can imagine conditions in which a clinician might impose an increasingly demanding swallowing adequacy requirement on thick liquid swallows. In this case, thickened liquids might earn a place in the list of rehabilitative techniques. A clinical book, however, is not the battleground for fighting classification battles. Therefore, our goal with the division into rehabilitative and compensatory is to classify them traditionally and by central tendencies. No division, including this one, is absolute, and certainly revisions in how methods are to be classified will occur. For now, however, here is how it seems to us.

LEE SILVERMAN VOICE THERAPY (LSVT)

Description of Method

This method of maximum performance training, which when introduced for the treatment of speech in men and women with Parkinson's disease (PD), emphasized the concept of "Think Loud," has now been introduced into swallowing treatment (El Sharkawi et al., 2002). Administering the treatment requires special training and certification. As a result, the method will be described only in brief detail here. Readers are cautioned that practicing the method on the basis of this description is prohibited. As will be demonstrated below, however, the method has promise as a treatment modality and, depending on one's practice, acquiring certification may well be worth it. Main steps/stages of the therapy are:

1. The method's essence is the exhortation and practice to be loud during production of progressively longer productions of "ah."
2. Another critical exercise is the increasingly competent and extended

production of pitch change on "ah" or its equivalent, from the lowest to the highest possible pitch.

3. Furthermore, the emphasis is on helping the patient learn to identify the physical and perceptual cues associated with increasingly competent performance.

4. The clinician's tasks are to explain, encourage, systematically increase the production requirements, evaluate patient performance, give suggestions for altering performance as necessary, and systematically move the patient toward ever more competent performance.

5. Counseling is critical because many patients question the mechanism of the treatment's effect on swallowing.

Modifications

The above is a bare bones description of the methodology. The required training will introduce clinicians to the subtleties, and they are many. Only a sampling, plus a brief discussion of an intensive amplitude of movement treatment (Farley, Fox, Ramig, & McFarland, in press), appear below.

1. Voice quality must be monitored so as not to allow harsh, strained phonation.

2. The emphasis must be on increasing respiratory drive as normally as possible and not on squeezing the larynx unnaturally to prolong phonation.

3. Determining the duration and pitch change targets requires approaching the maximum the patient is capable of without deterioration in quality or consistent loudness.

4. Farley et al. (in press) describe the development of a treatment that emphasizes not only getting louder but also making bigger reaching and walking movements. They are calling this treatment "Big and Loud." It, too, requires certification training. The essence of the method is that patients are given intensive practice in walking, reaching, and other daily tasks with greatly extended amplitudes. Early data are promising for speech and movement. Swallowing data are not apparently available.

Frequency and Duration

When used for speech, the prescription is for 16 sessions in 4 weeks with intensive homework. More, but seldom fewer, treatments may be necessary for dysphagic patients. Our dysphagia prescription is for a minimum of 16 weeks of home practice with one 1-hour clinic session scheduled every 1 or 2 weeks, depending on progress.

Candidacy

Those with PD would appear to be the best candidates; however, promising speech (swallow not evaluated) effects have also been reported for a limited number of patients with multisystem atrophy as well (Countryman & Ramig, 1994). We consider its use for all patterns of dysphagia in PD and in diagnoses where performance during swallowing seems generally underpowered or underdriven. Signs that may indicate this state (recognizing that other more focal conditions such as weakness may also produce similar signs) include slow bolus formation, delayed initiation of the pharyngeal swallow with bolus trickling more or less continuously into the pharynx prior to initiation, reduced opening of the upper esophageal sphincter (UES), and residuals throughout the swallowing track. Depending on pattern, as when inadequate airway protection is a prominent sign, we may add other swallowing-specific techniques to be practiced in tandem. Those will be described below.

Effects

The data from a small group of PD patients to be reviewed below suggests a positive effect on behavioral plasticity. Specifically, rocking of the bolus, initiation of the swallow, and amount of postswallow residue were all reduced, and airway protection was enhanced. Admittedly, the mechanism or mechanisms remain speculative, but activation of wider areas of nervous activity in the early days followed by a progressive narrowing of the locus of nervous system activity (when the method is used to improve speech) is the pattern of neural activation (Liotti et al., 2003). The result may be the same for swallowing, but that remains an experimental question. Increased awareness may also be an explanation at a psychological level. Muscle strengthening seems unlikely but endurance may be increased. In the right clinician's hands, a placebo effect can also be predicted and, along with increased neural activation, may explain early therapeutic effects.

The Evidence

At the time of this publication, a single study on swallowing effects in move- ment disorders, specifically PD, has been reported (El Sharkawi et al., 2002). As outlined above, LSVT is a promising treatment for dysphagia in PD that begs for further investigations.

RESPIRATORY MUSCLE STRENGTH TRAINING (RMST)

Description of Methods

RMST is of two main types: inspiratory (IMST) and expiratory (EMST). These two interacting respiratory muscle systems can be treated separately or simultaneously with resistance training. The training with the largest apparent effect requires the patient to forcefully inhale (IMST) or exhale (EMST) against graded, quantifiable resistance. A variety of commercial devices, such as that shown in Figure 14–1, are available for such training. Based on the amount of resistance provided, a certain amount of air pressure (measured in centimeters of water) is necessary to open the valve. If the resistance is systematically manipulated based on each patient's maximum strength, increased strength can be developed. Greater resistance and fewer repetitions are most effective for strength; less resistance and more repetitions may be more effective for endurance, although far less is known about appropriate prescriptions for endurance (Kays & Robbins, 2007). The methodology for strengthening as developed by Sapienza and colleagues (Kim & Sapienza, 2005; Saleem, Sapienza, & Okun, 2005; Sapienza, Davenport, & Martin, 2002; Silverman et al., 2006) is as follows.

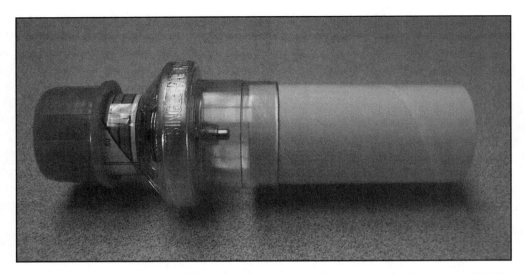

Figure 14–1. Expiratory threshold device for expiratory muscle strength training (EMST). Republished with permission of Aspire Products.

Measure maximum inspiratory (MIPs) and expiratory (MEPs) pressures using a digital pressure gauge meter such as that shown in Figure 14-2. An average of three maximum performance trials or an average of trials (regardless of number, though no more than eight should be elicited) that vary no more than 5% forms the basis of the calculation of normal, and if abnormal, it is the basis of the first calculation in determining the eventual training level.

If reduced, training begins with either an inspiratory or an expiratory pressure resistance of 75% of the average maximum pressure. Patient criteria for either inspiratory or expiratory training are specified in the Candidacy section. Table 14-1 shows normative data for maximum expiratory pressures compiled by Kim & Sapienza (2005). As clinicians, we admittedly know less about normative data for MIP than we do MEP. Dysphagia clinicians seeking this data will need to search the literature.

Introduce the treatment and the device to the patient. This step includes such common sense activities as describing how the device works and allowing patient to manipulate it. Place a nose clip on the patient to reduce nasal airflow. Begin a series of trials to orient the patient to inhaling or blowing into the device without allowing air to escape around the lips or out the nose. This usually means helping the patient learn to grip the device's mouthpiece tightly with teeth and lips, a requirement that often means considerable practice and perhaps selected procedural modifications (see below).

Instruct the patient to take a very deep breath. With inspiratory training, the valve will resist this inhalation until sufficient force is generated to open the valve. In expiratory training, the inhalation is taken, held, and then the device is positioned in the mouth prior to exhalation.

For expiratory training, once the patient has taken a deep breath and the device has been positioned, the next step

Ask frequent questions about any discomfort or light-headedness, especially in the beginning. If one or more of these side effects is reported, encourage patient rest between trials. If they return, reduce the resistance by 10% or so and try again. If training at any resistance causes side effects, then this method is not for that particular person. Once the proper resistance has been established, complete the schedule outlined in the section on duration and frequency.

Modifications

Seldom do methods work in the simplified way portrayed in publications. The entire complexity of this treatment is impossible to describe; however, certain common modifications are outlined below.

1. May have to begin by merely having a patient blow without resistance and then gradually introduce the device.
2. May have to have patient practice first with just the mouthpiece in place.
3. May have to manually provide buccal support to help patient maintain a lip seal around the device's mouthpiece. This need often disappears with training.
4. May have then to teach the patient/caregiver to use her own hand to provide this support while exhaling.
5. Nose clips may temporarily disrupt patient's coordination and require some practice coordinating blowing with the plug in place.
6. May have to spend extra time teaching patients to recognize the sound and feel of the valve breaking and to differentiate reduced pressure

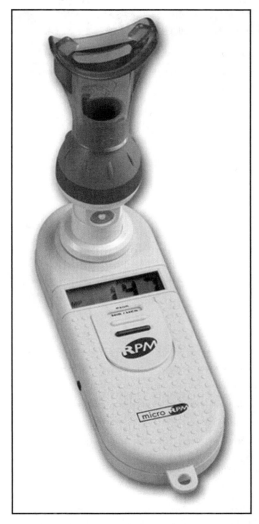

Figure 14–2. Digital pressure gauge meter for the measurement of maximum inspiratory and expiratory strength (MicroRPM). Republished with permission of Cardinal Health.

is to forcefully exhale into the device until the valve opens. Help the patient learn to identify the feel and sound of the valve opening. This step often requires multiple trials and can be hampered by hearing loss. For the hearing impaired, the cue to the valve's opening will need to be the air flow and resistance changes.

Table 14–1. Compilation of normative data for maximum expiratory pressures by age

Age Range	Ringqvist[1]		Black & Hyatt[2]		Chen & Kuo[3]		Enright et al.[4]		Berry et al.[5]	
	Men (n)	Women (n)	Men (n)	Women (n)*	Men (n)	Women (n)	Men (n)	Women (n)	Men (n)	Women (n)
18–29	247 ± 41 (37)	170 ± 29 (33)	—	—	141.2 ± 8.8 (20)	97.9 ± 5.4 (20)	—	—	—	—
30–39	248 ± 38 (12)	163 ± 29 (8)	—	—	136.6 ± 8.9 (20)[†]	92.8 ± 4.2 (20)[†]	—	—	—	—
40–49	253 ± 52 (15)	178 ± 33 (12)	—	—	—	—	—	—	—	—
50–59	252 ± 32 (13)	157 ± 28 (12)	218 ± 74 (5)	145 ± 40 (8)	133.6 ± 8.9 (20)[‡]	88.4 ± 6.2 (20)[‡]	—	—	—	—
60–64	209 ± 49 (16)[§]	157 ± 27 (17)[§]	209 ± 74 (3)	140 ± 40 (4)	117.4 ± 7.4 (20)[¶]	75.1 ± 5.1 (20)[¶]	—	—	—	—
65–69	—	—	197 ± 74 (7)	135 ± 40 (6)	—	—	188 (113)	125 (176)	190 ± 55[**] (44)	125 ± 36[**] (57)
70–74	200 ± 42 (13)	165 ± 29 (10)	185 ± 74 (10)	128 ± 40 (10)	—	—	179 (105)	121 (119)	—	—
75–79	—	—	—	—	—	—	161 (59)	102 (85)	—	—
80–84	—	—	—	—	—	—	142 (43)	84 (34)	—	—
85+	—	—	—	—	—	—	131 (9)	94 (13)	—	—

Note: Mean MEP or mean MEP ± standard deviation (in cm H_2O) included.

[1]Ringqvist T. The ventilatory capacity in healthy subjects. An analysis of causal factors with special reference to the respiratory forces. Scand J Clin Lab Invest Suppl. 1966;88:67.

[2]Black LF, Hyatt RE. Maximal respiratory pressures: Normal values and relationship to age and sex. Am Rev Respir Dis. 1969;99(5):698–99.

[3] Chen HI, Kuo CS. Relationship between respiratory muscle function and age, sex, and other factors. J Appl Physiol. 1989;66(2):945.

[4]Enright PL, Kronmal RA, Manolio TA, Schenker MB, Hyatt RE. Respiratory muscle strength in the elderly. Correlates and reference values. Cardiovascular Health Study Research Group. Am J Respir Crit Care Med. 1994;149(2 Pt 1):432.

[5]Berry JK, Vitalo CA, Larson JL, Patel M, Kim MJ. Respiratory muscle strength in older adults. Nurs Res. 1996;45(3):155. Linear regression for men, MEPs = 360 − 2.47 × age; for women, MEPs = 242 −1.75 × age.

*Number of subjects in each group in this column was not defined in original paper, so we estimated number of subjects from figure shown in published manuscript.

[†]Range of age = 31–45.

[‡]Range of age = 46–60.

[§]Range of age = 60–69.

[¶]Range of age = 61–75.

[**]Range of age = 65 and older.

Note. From "Implications of Expiratory Muscle Strength Training for Rehabilitation in the Elderly: Tutorial," Kim, J.,& Sapienza, C. M. (2005). *Journal of Rehabilitation Research and Development, 42,* pp. 211–224.

because of a broken lip seal from that of an opening valve.

7. May have to systematically change the interval between each trial to accommodate fatigue.

8. May have to change the resistance if patient cannot reach the 25 trial recommendation per day (see Frequency and Duration below).

9. May have to train someone to hold the device if patient has disabling tremor, dyskinesia, or weakness, or engage the assistance of a caregiver.

10. May have to go longer between adjustments or in total treatment time than is prescribed (see Frequency and Duration below). The criterion for making these decisions is failure for MIPs or MEPs to improve after a period of treatment.

Frequency and Duration

Frequency and duration for EMST have been worked out in PD. A *minimum* schedule of 25 trials per day, 6 days per week for 4 weeks, is required for an early effect resulting from neural activation and for a later strengthening effect. Increasing the duration beyond 4 weeks seems to be associated with further increases in strength (Saleem et al., 2005). The weaker a patient is, the longer the training duration is likely to be unless increased strength is impossible. Strength should be measured every 1 or at most 2 weeks. Recall that training used for strengthening is to be conducted at 75% of maximum inspiratory or expiratory pressure. For endurance training an intensified schedule of 50 to 100 trials per day for a minimum of 6 weeks at 40% of maximum pressure may be sufficient, although no data are available to support this recommendation.

Candidacy

PD is the movement disordered population for whom RMST has been demonstrated to have speech effects. In addition, one patient with a mixed ataxic-hyperkinetic-spastic dysarthria secondary to myoclonus, ataxia, and increased tone as part of Lance-Adams syndrome has also been successfully treated with EMST (Jones et al., 2006), and a treatment study in patients with atypical parkinsonian conditions is planned for patients with conditions such as multiple system atrophy (MSA) and progressive supranuclear palsy (PSP). Presumably, it will be demonstrated that EMST and IMST are appropriate for a wide variety of patients. Candidacy may be further widened for a treatment combining both forms of respiratory muscle strength training. Unfortunately, the only single device to allow both forms of strengthening is limited by poor calibration and training range.

The effect of RMST on swallowing is only now emerging in the literature. EMST has been shown to have a positive influence on swallowing (Wheeler, Chiara, & Sapienza, 2007) and coughing (Kim & Sapienza, 2005). Future research may show that EMST may be indicated for those with respiratory or other muscle system weakness (e.g., the suprahyoids) or decreased endurance. Such weakness can be measured in the expiratory muscles and inferred, albeit tentatively, in the suprahyoids from evaluation of anterior hyoid movement. Wheeler and colleagues (2007) specifically highlight reduced hyoid movement during swallowing as a criterion. Other patterns such as reduced laryngeal closure or pharyngeal peristalsis may be criteria as well, but the data are still unavailable.

Criteria for choosing whether to do IMST or EMST are not fully developed. Isolated diaphragmatic weakness would prompt IMST, but isolated weakness is rare in movement disorders. The relative amount of inhalatory and exhalatory muscle weakness could serve as a criterion, with the decision to treat the weaker component. Our experience in movement disorders is primarily with EMST. We often use it as a generalized treatment in response to the full range of oral and pharyngeal abnormalities, assuming some respiratory muscle weakness or reduced endurance can be demonstrated. Clinicians may also choose to combine it with more specific swallowing-related activities and even compensatory approaches.

Effects

Placebo, neural activation, strengthening, and endurance effects may all be expected from this method. Combining IMST and EMST may increase all these effects but that experiment has not been done, and the effects reported are primarily for EMST alone. EMST may improve function of respiratory and submental musculature (Wheeler et al., 2007), as well as lingual, velopharyngeal, pharyngeal, and laryngeal musculature. This has not been demonstrated experimentally. Increased respiratory muscle strength or endurance may also improve cough. Increased extent of hyolaryngeal movement and UES opening because of improved submental muscle activity, improved lingual propulsion of bolus, improved velopharyngeal valving, improved movement of bolus through the pharynx, and improved airway protection may also occur because of the method's impact on strength or endurance of these muscle systems.

The Evidence

Evidence for the therapeutic effect of EMST is beginning to accumulate. EMST for 20 weeks resulted in a 158% gain in maximum expiratory pressure (MEP) for a 54-year-old female with a 5-year history of PD (Saleem et al., 2005). After 4 weeks without training, her MEPs had decreased 16% but remained 104% above pretraining levels. Interestingly, her Unified Parkinson's Disease Rating Scale (UPDRS) score also improved between weeks 4 and 20. However, unlike MEP, the UPDRS returned to baseline after the 4-week no-treatment period. Nonetheless, the possibility of generalization of treatment effect cannot be ignored. Silverman and colleagues (2006) provide additional information on three patients with IPD treated for 4 weeks. All three had large increases in MEPs with increases of 91.3%, 75.3%, and 79.5%. Although inspiratory muscles were not simultaneously trained, MIPs

also increased. Swallowing was not measured. Regarding swallowing, Wheeler et al. (2007) studied the effect on EMST in 20 healthy participants and found increased motor unit recruitment of the submental muscles following training, which may very well have implications for individuals with dysphagia.

LINGUAL STRENGTHENING

Description of Methods

Because of the tongue's importance to bolus preparation and initiating the entire chain of swallowing events, treatments for it have been of interest for decades. This section will not include a review of these earlier and for the most part inadequately motivated and data- and concept-starved efforts, most of which are grouped under the rubric of oral motor exercises. Instead, the focus here will be on an instrumental treatment for tongue strengthening, the Iowa Oral Performance Instrument (IOPI) (Robin, Goel, Somodi, & Luschei, 1992; Robin, Somodi, & Luschei, 1991). Clinicians, of course, can employ other available and soon to be developed devices for lingual strengthening, such as the Madison Oral Strengthening Therapeutic (MOST) device (Hewitt et al., 2008). Indeed, a section on modifications will describe some of these possibilities.

The methodology to be described will be one approach used with the IOPI (Figure 14–3). For the present discussion, the critical components of this device are an air-filled tongue bulb, as seen in Figure 14–4, connected to a pressure transducer, which is in turn connected to an amplifier, signal conditioner, and digital voltmeter. The tongue bulb is posi-

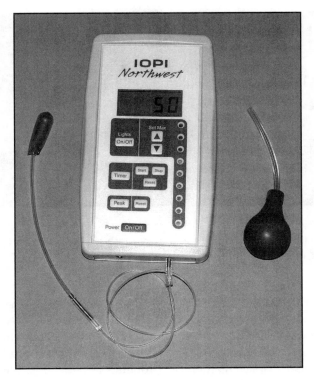

Figure 14–3. The Iowa Oral Performance Instrument (IOPI) shown with tongue and hand bulbs. Republished with permission of IOPI Northwest Co. LLC.

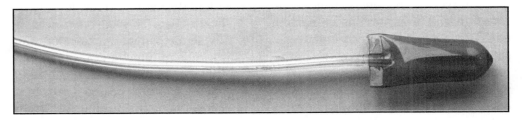

Figure 14–4. The Iowa Oral Performance Instrument (IOPI) tongue bulb. Republished with permission of IOPI Northwest Co. LLC.

tioned in the mouth either anteriorly or posteriorly, and the squeezing activity of the tongue against the hard palate is registered as a change in pressure measured in kilopascals (kPa). As shown in Figure 14-5, the tongue bulb can also be adapted to measure lateral tongue strength. Pressure can also activate a light display by turning a column of light from red to green. The amount of pressure necessary to change these colors can be set by the clinician so that greater or lesser pressure is necessary. This arrangement allows a form of knowledge

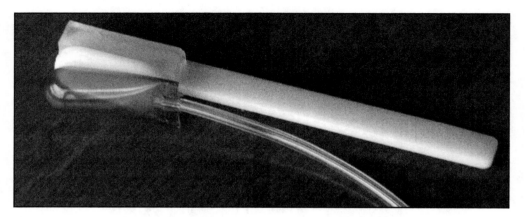

Figure 14–5. The tongue bulb of the Iowa Oral Performance Instrument (IOPI) adapted for measurement of lateral tongue strength. Republished with permission of IOPI Northwest Co. LLC.

of performance (KP) for the patient. Failure to turn the light from red to green signals inadequate upward lingual pressure against the bulb, for example. Pressure in kPas is also displayed, thereby heightening the amount of knowledge the patient receives.

The IOPI is both a diagnostic and a therapeutic device. Diagnostically, it will provide quantification of maximum lingual pressure a patient can generate anteriorly and posteriorly. As a treatment tool, progressively greater pressure targets (as a surrogate for strength) can be provided in a standardized strengthening paradigm. It is traditional to measure endurance as well by requiring a patient to hold a target that is 50% of maximum pressure for as long as possible. As will be documented in the section on data, both activities are justified by observations of the relationships among signs of abnormal swallowing and reductions in pressure (or strength). Conceptually, the motivations are that IOPI (and other similar instruments available or under development) allows quantification and satisfies the criterion of specificity. Train-

ing can occur during swallowing. This contrasts markedly with traditional oral exercises where patients are directed to protrude or otherwise move their tongues as far as possible or to protrude and resist the pressure of the clinician's effort to push the tongue back into the mouth with a tongue blade. A generic methodology follows:

1. Orient the patient to the device and the treatment. This step often includes having the patient practice performing the requested target on multiple occasions and may also require frequent cueing, repeated trials, and repositioning by the clinician. Often this step can consume much of a session, but it is critical if the treatment is to have a chance at success.

2. Determine whether the potential patient has a reduction in lingual pressure during maximum performance testing of the anterior and posterior tongue. Robbins and colleagues (1995, 2005, 2007) identify abnormally reduced pressure as being below a value of 40 kPa, pre-

sumably as an average of five or so trials. They positioned the tongue at the anterior site 10 mm back from the tongue tip; the posterior site is defined in their work as 10 mm anterior to the "most posterior circumvallate papilla" (Robbins et al., 2007, p. 151). The key here is to record the pressure that is most consistently generated plus or minus 5%. A common command is, "Push the bulb against the roof of your mouth as hard as you can." This can be the methodology for determining candidacy and for setting the training pressures.

3. An alternative method for determining the pressure to be initially used in treatment is to accept as maximum the highest pressure in six trials completed in two sets of three. Training then occurs at 75% of that maximum.

4. Measure endurance by having patient hold a pressure that is 50% of maximum for as long as possible. Lazarus and colleagues (2000) recommend a 2-minute interval between all trials.

5. To train swallowing pressure (strength) of lingual elevation in the absence of a swallow, set the target at approximately 75% of maximum.

6. Begin a series of five or so consecutive trials with an appropriate rest interval between. Appropriateness will be determined as a pattern of responses that produces a variable pattern of success but not one characterized by successively greater pressure reductions. The goal is that the patient train hard but successfully. An alternative is having the patient complete as many successive swallows at the target pressure as possible. If more than 8 to 12 successive, successful repetitions are possible, the pressure target is probably set too low.

7. Repeat (see Frequency and Duration section below).

Modifications

As noted before, a standard protocol for this method's use is still being developed. Therefore, multiple experimental modifications are ongoing. In this section, we will list some for consideration.

One option for testing and treating is to measure maximum tongue pressure during swallowing (as opposed to a non-swallowing task of merely pushing the tongue to the tip of the mouth) in response to the command, "Push the bulb against the roof of your mouth as hard as you can and swallow." In this option the patient is instructed to swallow dry but to swallow as hard as possible. A 2-minute interval between each of five or so trials can be employed, especially if successive values are declining or if variability is greater than 5%. The usual pattern is that the second and third trials are greater than the first, after which performance may get more variable. Three consecutive values within 5% of one another can be used to determine maximum strength and endurance, and the mean of these can be taken as the "score."

An option to presetting the anterior and posterior sites for training is to identify sites anteriorly and posteriorly where the highest pressures are generated during swallowing. Probably, but not inevitably, the sites chosen using this method will approximate the predetermined ones.

Sometimes only one site can be trained because of difficulty with positioning or maintaining the bulb in a similar place from trial to trial.

An alternative to strengthening at approximately 75% of maximum effort during the entire treatment is to follow the Robbins et al. (2007) guideline and train at 60% during week one and at 80% from then on. This paradigm, as developed in stroke patients, requires 8 weeks of treatment. If a person's maximum strength (pressure) reaches normal limits earlier, then treatment can be discontinued. If progress continues between testing periods and if resources are available to support continued training, continuing to train until progress stops or until a normal range is reached is also appropriate.

Training can also be done with other devices. For example, the KayPENTAX Digital Swallowing Workstation allows the use of two- and three-bulb arrays as shown in Figure 14–6 and Figure 14–7. This treatment arrangement allows training during swallowing more readily than does the IOPI, because the strip of three transducers is affixed to the palate with an adhesive such as Stomahesive. The anterior can be positioned just posterior to the alveolar ridge. The training paradigm can be identical to that used with the IOPI.

Another modification may be to simply use a tongue blade. Lazarus and colleagues (2003) reported no significant difference in posttreatment strength after home practice 5 of 7 days per week for 4 weeks. In this study, participants practiced five sets of 10 repetitions of maximum strength training.

Frequency and Duration

The paradigm worked out for stroke can be a useful guideline. Robbins and colleagues (2007) treated for 8 weeks. Frequency was 30 repetitions per day for the anterior site and the posterior site, divided

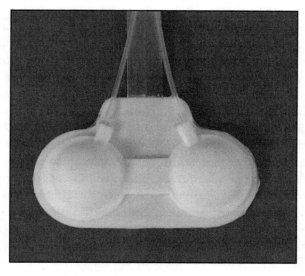

Figure 14–6. Two-bulb lingual pressure transducer to be used with the KayPENTAX Digital Swallowing Workstation. Published with the permission of KayPENTAX.

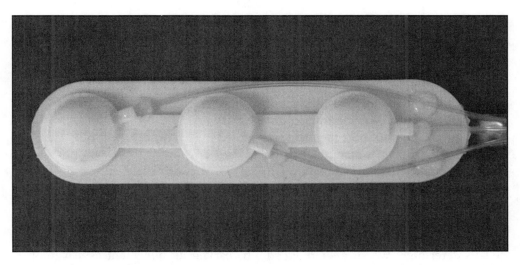

Figure 14–7. Three-bulb lingual transducer array to be used with the KayPENTAX Digital Swallowing Workstation. Published with the permission of KayPENTAX.

into groups of 10. Training was completed 3 days per week. Testing to determine if the pressure-training target could be increased was done every 2 weeks.

We regard this as a minimum schedule and recommend training 6 of 7 days per week with weekly reevaluation. Also, twice the number of repetitions per day if the patient can manage may heighten the treatment's effects but, of course, the data allowing us to know this for sure are yet unavailable. If strength is improving, and if resources to support it are available, treatment can continue, particularly if functional effects occur. If, however, the swallow is not improving despite substantial strength increases, the clinician should reevaluate the hypothesis about lingual strength being the explanation for dysphagia.

Effects

Early and later effects even in the same swallowing sign may have different bases.

The earliest effects are probably related to the placebo effect and to increased neural activation or recruitment of larger portions of the central nervous system network capable of contributing to performance in tongue strength. Later effects may well be improved strength (or endurance), accomplished by muscle hypertrophy, as well as possible other fiber and cellular changes. With increased lingual strength *may* come improved oral stage performance, such as bolus formation and movement, as well as changes in pharyngeal stage signs. Data from stroke subjects suggests that improved pressure generation during swallowing may result in better airway protection as signaled by improved scores on the Penetration-Aspiration Scale (PAS), reduced pharyngeal residue, increased pharyngeal response time, decreased oral transit duration, and improved domains of quality of life as measured by SWAL-QOL (Robbins et al., 2007). Additionally, lingual muscle hypertrophy was observed in some patients.

Candidacy

Candidates are those patients with deficits in strength or endurance that appear to explain one or more serious signs of dysphagia. Unfortunately, determining these relationships depends on clinical experience. Sign that help support the logic are difficulties with lingual manipulation of the bolus, poor movement and control of the bolus, premature spillage of the bolus into the pharynx, and vallecular residue in a person with reduced tongue strength. Endurance is even more difficult to determine. We suspect reduced endurance when patients tell us they fatigue during a meal, have more problems toward the end than at the beginning of a meal, and, of course, show reduced endurance on testing. Fortunately, data do exist showing reduced lingual strength in PD (Solomon, Robin, Lorell, Rodnitzky, & Luschei, 1994; Solomon, Robin, & Luschei, 2000). The relationship of that weakness to swallowing disorders must be established for individual patients, not only in PD, but in the other movement disorders as well.

The Evidence

Data are available for normal elderly and for a small group of stroke patients. Of special interest in this section is that in the elderly, tongue strengthening in the nonswallowing treatment paradigm was accompanied by increased lingual pressures during swallowing (Robbins et al., 2005). Most of the stroke data have been reviewed at appropriate places above to support rough guidelines about how the treatment is to be done and what its potential effects are. For the stroke subjects, improvements in swallowing pressures, amount of postswallow residue, selected durational measures, penetration-aspiration performance, and selected domains of quality of life (QoL) have been documented (Robbins et al., 2007).

MENDELSOHN MANEUVER

Description of Method

The Mendelsohn maneuver's aim is to enhance superior and especially anterior hyolaryngeal movement as a way of increasing the duration and extent of UES opening during the swallow. This technique was first documented by Logemann and Kahrilas in 1990. Interestingly enough, when we began to write this section, we realized we did not know the origin of the name of the Mendelsohn maneuver. J. A. Logemann responded to our query and reported that a research assistant and medical student, Martin Mendelsohn, was pivotal in the development of this technique and accordingly it was named after him. Mendelsohn later finished his medical training and is now an otolaryngologist practicing in Australia (personal communication, April 18, 2008).

In its simplest form, the method's steps are:

1. The clinician explains the method, beginning with the notion that it requires initiating a swallow, trying to stop the swallow at the point when the hyolaryngeal complex is at its maximum excursion for 2 seconds, and then completing the swallow.
2. The clinician demonstrates the movement, having the patient place a hand or fingers on the clinician's larynx while the maneuver is executed.

3. Repeat as many times with as much explanation as is necessary.
4. Next, the patient and clinician lightly touch the patient's larynx during performance of the maneuver.
5. Repeat, with the clinician giving verbal knowledge of performance (KP) in the form of specific observations about why the patient's execution was adequate or not.
6. Continue practicing until the patient can perform the activity a minimum of 80% of the time without having to feel the larynx.
7. Rest between trials and repeat.

Modifications

This complex maneuver allows a variety of modifications, most of which will be familiar to experienced clinicians. Only what may be the most important are described below.

Logemann and Kahrilas's (1990) original instruction was to swallow normally, and when the patient feels her voice box elevate, she was to grab it with her throat muscles for a count of three before relaxing.

A rough strengthening paradigm can be created in an effort to improve strength by applying digital resistance to the elevation of the hyoid. No report of this variation is available; thus the procedure is nonstandardized. The notion is, however, that a patient can be taught to use a finger to resist upward movement of the larynx. "Stronger" movement may result. A more quantifiable method for enhancing activity is described in the following paragraph.

Surface electromyography (sEMG), derived from electrodes placed over the suprahyoid muscles under the chin, can be used to set muscle activity targets and provide knowledge of results (KR) in the form of muscle activity. Using sEMG in this way is a specialized skill. Interested clinicians can read about the method in Crary (1995), Crary and colleagues (2004), and Huckabee and Cannito (1999).

Frequency and Duration

No data are available, and therefore the clinician is forced to rely on general principles. If the aim is to simply increase neural drive, then a few (perhaps as few as three) closely spaced sessions may be sufficient. If strengthening or skill training is the goal, then other considerations arise. Intensive practice should be performed for a minimum of 6 weeks at a frequency of 6 out of 7 days per week. A minimum of 25 repetitions per day, with three to four times that number being better, would seem an appropriate prescription, although more is probably better. For strengthening, the additional requirement is to systematically increase the load. Increasing endurance may well require systematically more trials per day for more than 6 weeks.

Much of this practice can be done at home, but the clinician would do well to see the patient at least once weekly to guarantee that increased skill, strength, or endurance is occurring.

When sEMG feedback is used, the frequency and duration data in two published reports differ extensively. Crary (1995) used daily treatments for 3 weeks to 7 months. It appears that other behavioral treatments continued after those times. Huckabee and Cannito (1999) used 2 hours of treatment daily for 5 days. Some of their patients also had additional traditional treatment with a professional, whereas others completed home programs. The variability in these data makes a single conclusion impossible, with the exception, perhaps, that the required frequency and duration are likely to differ not only for different therapeutic aims, but for different patients.

Effects

The placebo effect from this exercise is unlikely to be obvious in the swallowing physiology, but patients may report the sensation of an improved swallow. Done correctly over time, this method can increase superior-anterior hyolaryngeal movement, with a resulting increase in the extent and duration of UES opening. Functionally, the effect may be that greater amounts of increasingly difficult boluses, such as meat, can pass through the UES and into the esophagus. It may also improve coordination of swallow events (Lazarus, Logemann, & Gibbons, 1993). The explanation for such changes early on in treatment may be increased neural activation. Later on, these results may result from strengthening of suprahyoid musculature or from increased endurance, depending on the paradigm.

Candidacy

The Mendelsohn maneuver is an option for patients whose UES opening is reduced in extent or duration. These reductions can be judged perceptually or measured exactly. Extent of UES opening in the adult is influenced by bolus size. For adults, the mean in centimeters for a 3 cc bolus is 0.51 (SD = 0.15). For a 20 cc bolus, an amount that more nearly approximates what adults swallow, the mean is 0.89 cm (SD = 0.28) (Leonard, Kendall, McKenzie,

Goncalves, & Walker, 2000). Other signs that may suggest candidacy for this approach include residuals in the pyriform sinuses after the swallow and reduced anterior movement of the hyoid. Normal anterior movement differs by gender and bolus size. For women swallowing a 3 cc bolus, the mean anterior movement is 1.62 cm (SD = 0.56). For a 20 cc bolus, this movement is 1.81 cm (SD = 0.73). For males swallowing a 3 cc bolus, the mean anterior hyolaryngeal movement is 2.12 cm (SD = 0.69), and this increases to 2.47 cm (SD = 0.68) for a 20 cc bolus (Leonard et al., 2000). Clinical acumen is necessary to separate impaired opening as a primary sign from impaired opening because of weak propulsion of the bolus from the mouth or from incoordination of multiple structures critical to the normal swallow.

The Evidence

Somewhat remarkably given this method's popularity, the data in support of a treatment effect are extremely limited. Logemann and Kahrilas (1990) initially studied this technique in a single patient following stroke, and this method was later studied in a small group of normal participants using videofluoroscopic swallow examination (VFSE) (Kahrilas, Logemann, Krugler, & Flanagan, 1991). Lazarus and colleagues (1993, 2002) have studied this approach in a limited number of head and neck cancer patients. Robbins and Levine (1993) described this approach in two patients with brainstem stroke who also had an accompanying myotomy. When KP is provided via sEMG, however, the data are more extensive and promising, though stroke, not movement disorders, is the diagnosis most often studied. Both Crary (1995) and Huck-abee and Cannito (1999) report changes in swallowing physiology and a high probability of a return to oral nutrition for tube-fed stroke patients. It is important to note that the sEMG was paired with a variety of behavioral treatments and not merely the Mendelsohn maneuver in these studies.

SHAKER HEAD RAISE

Description of Method

This method was developed to enhance UES opening by strengthening the supra-hyoid musculature primarily responsible for hyolaryngeal elevation and subsequent UES opening (Shaker et al., 1997; Shaker et al., 2002). It was reasoned that raising the head while lying supine would strengthen that musculature. In its purest form, this method requires the following procedures.

The patient is helped to assume a supine posture with the shoulder blades and buttocks in contact with a supportive surface. Once positioned, a series of three 1-minute head lifts, each followed by 1 minute of rest, is performed. The patient elevates the head sufficiently to allow visualization of the feet. Next, the patient performs 30 head lifts without the extended duration of holding this posture.

Modifications

Data on the method's effect, to be reviewed below, are available only for the purest form of the method and are not available for patients with movement disorders. In our experience, however, many patients are initially not capable of performing the method as described. Several modifications are logical, although it is to be emphasized that data on effect are unavailable.

The first is to reduce the number of repetitions in each series. The second is to increase the rest period between groups of trials. The third is to reduce the duration of the lift on the three 1-minute trials. A more radical alteration is to reduce the angle by having the patient sit upright in a recliner-style chair to begin the exercise, and then increase the angle as performance improves. No specific guidelines for angle increase are available, but patient performance can be a guide. The goal would be to systematically approximate the ideal form of the exercise or achieve the outcome of an improved swallow despite the angle.

Another modification, and one consistent with the spirit of strengthening principles, would be to position the patient at the steepest angle consistent with acceptable performance and then gradually add resistance by attaching soft weights to the head. In this modification, the load the patient must lift is systematically increased.

Frequency and Duration

Effects derived from head and neck cancer and stroke patients were achieved with three sessions per day, every day for 6 weeks. Probably for most patients this frequency and duration are a minimum, especially if any of the angle variations are used, although systematic assessment by whatever means are appropriate may be a better guide to frequency and duration beyond the minimum of 6 weeks, which is an arbitrary endpoint.

Simply increasing neural drive to the suprahyoid musculature with a short bout of treatment does not seem to make sense because of the treatment's aim of strengthening.

Strengthening would seem to require, at a minimum, reaching the 90 repetitions of the head raise with no hold at the top and the nine 1-minute holds per day, 6 days out of every 7, as a minimum. Increased strength could be posited for those who start below this target and then are able systematically to reach it. For those who start at the 90 repetitions level, improved strength would seem to require adding resistance, as described under Modifications.

Increased endurance might require a larger number of repetitions per day in a less than supine position, but this is purely speculative.

Candidacy

A number of signs and presumed underlying pathophysiology determine candidacy. However, there are contraindications as well; foremost among them is that patients with problems of the cervical spine should not be prescribed this technique. Indications for the method are outlined below.

The method appears to be most promising for patients with inadequate UES opening because of reduced anterior hyolaryngeal movement. Consistently reduced UES opening in the presence of good bolus propulsion, reduced anterior hyoid movement, and no reason to suspect the patency of UES opening are criteria for introducing a strengthening paradigm. That same pattern, with the exception that fatigue or lack of endurance is suggested by adequate early and inadequate later UES opening, supports the decision for an endurance paradigm.

Reduced opening of the UES because of fibrotic or other tissue abnormalities may also respond to the method. Of course, these changes are not part of the pathophysiology of the movement disorders.

This may be the method of choice in cases where the UES opening is narrowed by Zenker's diverticulum or osteophytes.

Presumed weakness in the suprahyoid musculature principally responsible for pulling the hyolaryngeal complex upward and forward makes the method logical as well.

Increased tone (spasticity and rigidity) and limited range of movement in those muscles are also criteria.

The need to compensate for inadequate movement of the bolus through the pharynx and UES because of inadequate lingual propulsion and initiation of the pharyngeal response may also be a criterion. However, treatment of the tongue would need to be tried first in all but those instances where a clinician is trying multiple methods simultaneously in the hopes of relatively quick improvements.

Effects

The major effect of a successful treatment is improved anterior excursion of the hyoid and opening of UES during swallowing, elimination of aspiration, and resumption of oral nutrition. These physiologic changes have not been documented in movement disorders. It is unknown if either strength or endurance is the basis for the improved UES activity. Nor are nervous system changes documented. Because the method does not require swallowing, it is less likely that functional changes result from the placebo or neural activation effects than for some other exercises. Nonetheless, both may well have at least some influence over early swallowing change because patients know the exercise is intended to improve swallowing.

The Evidence

Three studies, two of normal individuals (Shaker et al., 1997; Alfonso, Ferdjallah, Shaker, & Wertsch, 1998) and one of patients with dysphagia secondary to neurogenic disease or head/neck cancer (Shaker et al., 2002), are the source of effect data for this exercise. In the study involving those with neurogenic dysphagia, the main outcome was change in type of nutrition. The results are promising, as the majority of patients were able to change from tube to oral nutrition. In the studies of normal subjects, the outcome was derived from sEMG, and the amplitude of signal was used as a surrogate for increased strength. Its inadequacy to that task was not discussed and need not distract us here. What the data show is greater neural activity of the supraglottic musculature, which is the aim of the treatment.

SUPRAGLOTTIC SWALLOW AND ITS VARIATIONS

Description of the Method

The essence of the method is to enhance laryngeal valving using Valsalva's maneuver to protect the airway during swallowing. A variety of techniques or at least

directions are or may be involved in this technique, which some writers divide into the supraglottic and super-supraglottic swallow. For example, Logemann (1991) describes the instructions for the *supraglottic swallow*: "The patient is instructed (a) to inhale and hold the breath at the top of the inhalation, (b) to swallow while holding the breath, and (c) after the swallow, to cough to clear any residual material" (p. 274). In contrast, with the *super-supraglottic swallow*, the same procedures are followed with increased "effort of the breath holding prior to the swallow . . . (to pull) the arytenoids cartilages forward to the base of the epiglottis and (close) the laryngeal entry at the level of the false vocal folds" (Logemann, 1991, p. 274). For many clinicians, including us, distinctions between these approaches are subtle and we will therefore collect these laryngeal closing approaches into one. By doing so, we recognize that the amount of effort, and therefore the physiologic consequences, may differ. Our procedure is generally as follows.

1. Urge the patient to forcibly approximate the vocal folds, preferably by envisioning the quick lifting of a very heavy object and then by producing an audible, sharp grunt.
2. Breath holding is encouraged at this point.
3. Next, the patient is urged to swallow hard.
4. The swallow is followed by a brisk throat clear or cough.
5. This is followed by a repeat swallow.
6. Finally, a brisk exhalation occurs.
7. If successful, the above steps are repeated.
8. A bolus is not mandatory. If a bolus is employed, it is often best to make it small and have it in place on the

tongue prior to the inhalation, which should be completed through the nose.

This method is deceptively difficult because tight laryngeal closure is difficult to judge clinically. For that reason, we urge patients to grunt forcibly during exhalation and then hold their breath as the most reliable sign of laryngeal closure. Simply telling a person to hold her breath is likely to be unsuccessful because that instruction may merely result in a person's ceasing to breathe, rather than the effortful breath hold with the larynx adducted that dysphagia clinicians are seeking.

Modifications

This is an extremely complex swallowing method. A variety of modifications are possible. Some may make the maneuver more successful; others are designed to simplify it for those with respiratory or cognitive impairment. Breath hold can be at the end of inhalation or after a brief exhalation. Somewhat remarkably, some patients seem to do better with a *less* rather than *more* effortful breath hold. Inhalation and exhalation can be through the nose or mouth; however, through the nose is better if a bolus is being used. The maneuver can be accomplished with or without a bolus and is probably best introduced without foods or liquids. The bolus can be introduced before or after the breath hold. The sequence can be shortened by eliminating all but the first three steps. Closure of the larynx can be facilitated by Valsalva's maneuver, during which, for example, the patient pulls up forcibly against the bottom of a chair during the breath hold.

Candidacy

Based on signs and assumed underlying pathophysiology, this method is most appropriate for:

1. Those with inadequate laryngeal valving either before or during the swallow because of reductions in strength or endurance.
2. Those with delayed laryngeal closure because of a reduction in strength or endurance, and who, for whatever reason, have large pharyngeal residuals after the swallow.
3. Movement disorders patients whose swallow is too fast (which is to say they propel the bolus into the pharynx prior to laryngeal closure) may also benefit.

Patients with significant respiratory or cognitive problems usually cannot comply with the complex set of steps; hence the simplifications. In addition, the method may require too long an apneic period for those with critical levels of respiratory compromise. A physician should be aware of and approve this methodology because it can be physically challenging. Generally, it is ill advised for those with coronary heart disease.

Frequency and Duration

No data are available. Therefore, these variables must be derived from other literature based on the clinician's intent. As a compensation, once the method is learned, the patient merely needs to practice it on every swallow or at least on every swallow of a material know to be a risk. The supraglottic swallow is a skill. For a patient to learn it, intensive practice with high repetition across several days may be necessary. Equally necessary will be active evaluation of adequacy of performance by the clinician and a systematic fading of KP by the clinician so that the patient learns to judge performance adequacy. Principles of behaviorial plasticity (see Chapter 11), in other words, need to be employed. It is our impression that clinicians either give up on the patient's learning prematurely or mistakenly assume that a few correct performances in the clinic predict correct performance outside the clinic.

Endurance may increase with a high number of repetitions, 6 of 7 days over a month or even more. Whether or not the method can be used to strengthen is an experimental question. Given the lack of resistance during the training, a substantive change in strength is probably not to be expected.

Effects

Physiologically, the effect may be to increase approximation of the arytenoids and epiglottis and enhance the closure of both false and true folds (Logemann, 1991). In a study of three head and neck cancer patients, Lazarus and colleagues (2002) documented increased tongue base and posterior pharyngeal wall pressure and reduced pharyngeal residual.

The Evidence

No data on those with movement disorders is extant, at least not to our knowledge. The data that do exist are for small groups of head and neck cancer and stroke patients and, for the most part, are not collected over a long period of time (Bulow et al., 1999, 2002; Lazarus et al., 1993). Presumably, they measure the effects of increased neural activation. The clinician is urged to use this method with care.

MASAKO MANEUVER

Description of Method

Fujiu, Logemann, and Pauloski (1995) observed a spontaneous increase in posterior pharyngeal wall excursion in patients following base of tongue resection. Based on this observation, Fujiu and Logemann (1996) developed a maneuver designed to mimic this increased pharyngeal wall activity in individuals with an intact base of tongue. Thus, the *Masako maneuver* (also known as the *tongue holding maneuver*) was born. The approach is simple to describe but often difficult to accomplish without considerable practice and guidance, sometimes including refinement in the requirements. The critical steps are:

1. Clinician instructs the patient to protrude tongue beyond the teeth.
2. The tongue is then anchored by the patient's gently biting down against the surface of the tongue, or, more frequently, the patient, clinician, or caregiver gently grasps the tongue tip with a gauze pad.
3. Once anchored, the patient is instructed to swallow. Sometimes the patient will struggle to swallow for several seconds before actually doing so.
4. If successful, the tongue is released and retracted.

5. After an appropriate pause for saliva to return to the mouth, the above steps are repeated.
6. The Masako maneuver should not be completed with food or liquid boluses.

Modifications

This relatively straightforward method predictably allows few modifications. The amount of protrusion is the most frequent modification. Some patients simply cannot swallow with the tongue fully protruded. In that case, the clinician clinically manipulates the amount of protrusion until the target is reached. The goal is for the patient to be able to swallow, but with effort. Subsequent goals are to encourage progressively more protrusion until maximum protrusion is reached or until the point is reached where a patient cannot swallow regardless of effort.

Tongue anchoring may have to become the responsibility of a caregiver for any patient unable to hold the tongue. Providing even a bit of moisture before each trial may facilitate the swallow. Special attention to helping a patient know that a complete swallow and not merely a heroic effort has occurred may also be necessary. Both the sound of swallow and the action of the hyolaryngeal complex can provide guidance.

Effects

A successful sequence of Masako swallows is calculated to increase posterior pharyngeal wall movement. Whether it has an effect on the tongue is undocumented. Certainly, placebo and neural activation effects can be posited, assuming a patient is capable of even the least challenging form of the method. Strength and endurance can also be increased at least theoretically, although whether this occurs in the tongue, posterior pharyngeal wall, or both remains to be seen. A modest increase in skill can also be postulated.

If, for whatever reason, the posterior pharyngeal wall begins moving anteriorly toward the tongue, a variety of positive influences on bolus flow may be expected. These include:

1. Improved valving of the palate so that material is less likely to enter the nose during the swallow.
2. Improved lingual initiation of the swallow, with possible influences on timing and completeness of the remainder of the swallow sequence.

Candidacy

As discussed above, this method was originally derived from observations in patients following tongue base resection, in whom increased posterior pharyngeal wall movement was observed. The goal of the maneuver was to enhance posterior pharyngeal movement to compensate for reduced posterior tongue movement in individuals without surgical resection. The concept is that enhanced anterior movement of the posterior pharyngeal wall in the form of a bulging superior pharyngeal constrictor could compensate for reduced posterior movements of the tongue.

For those with movement disorders, the best candidates are therefore those with inadequate approximation of posterior tongue to posterior pharyngeal wall during the swallow. The method can be combined with others known to enhance tongue movement or if such methods have failed.

Frequency and Duration

No data on frequency and duration have been published; therefore, the clinician must rely on general guidelines. Presumably, the placebo effect and increased neural activation can be expected for the tongue and pharynx after only a few repetitions. Secondarily, if completed with sufficient load (i.e., swallowing while tongue is anchored), the exercise can lead to strengthening of the tongue. If strengthening is the goal, then maximum tongue protrusion and a minimum of 5 or 6 weeks of treatment, 6 days per week, and at least 25 repetitions per day is a minimum appropriate schedule. The more severe the problem, the greater the frequency and duration that may be necessary for maximum effects. Endurance may increase with less or equal tongue protrusion and a greater number of trials per day.

The Evidence

The data are thus far limited to individuals with intact swallow function. In these 10 normal participants, increased bulging of the posterior pharyngeal wall was observed (Fujiu & Logemann, 1996).

SHOWA MANEUVER

Description of Method

The Showa maneuver was developed at the Showa Hospital in Japan by Hirano and colleagues (1999). This technique involves the following steps:

1. Firmly hold breath.
2. Press the tongue forcibly up and back against the hard palate while continuing to maintain a firm breath hold.
3. Swallow as hard as possible, while forcibly contracting all the muscles of face, throat, and neck.
4. Release breath hold.
5. Repeat.

Modifications

Although more complex than the Masako maneuver, only a few modifications of this method seem logical:

1. Having the patient forcibly grunt as described in the supraglottic swallow may be a useful refinement.
2. The direction to press the tongue upward and backward against the hard palate may result in a static posture not leading to a swallow. Therefore, we often change the direction to one that encourages movement, such as, "Push your tongue up and back against the roof of your mouth as you swallow." We then add the part about contracting all the muscles in the face, mouth, and neck.
3. Step 2 may be eliminated altogether.
4. Steps 1 and 4 can be deleted, in which case the maneuver becomes the simplest form of the hard swallow (see below).

Candidacy

No data on the method's use in movement disorders has been published. The sign and pathophysiology that may justify the method's use are inadequate posterior-superior movement of the tongue when initiating the swallow because of weakness or poor endurance, leading in turn to:

1. Slow, inadequate movement of the bolus through the pharynx and into the UES.
2. Large amounts of pharyngeal residue, perhaps especially in the valleculae.
3. Reduced laryngeal valving before or during the swallow because of strength, endurance, or coordination impairment.
4. Possible reduced duration and extent of UES opening during the swallow because of inadequacies in initial swallowing initiation timing or power.

Effects

This method, which combines elements of both the hard swallow and the supraglottic swallow, may effect both initiation of the swallow by vigorous tongue action and airway closure during the swallow. Presumably this method does not strengthen musculature, although this remains an experimental question. Its influence may result from the placebo effect and neural activation, in which recruitment of a more expansive network of nervous system control of swallowing occurs than is present in the untreated swallow. It may also be seen as a skill-building task in that many patients improve in its performance. If this is true, then it might be expected that a more permanent expansion of cortical and subcortical neural substrates of swallowing control develops. Endurance may also increase with the right frequency and duration of practice.

Frequency and Duration

No frequency and duration information is available, so the clinician must again rely on general principles. A limited number of sessions with 25 or so repetitions per session may be enough to achieve both placebo and neural activation effects. Skill and endurance (especially endurance) will usually take more repetitions for more sessions. Intensive practice for a minimum of 6 weeks, at a frequency of 6 out of 7 days, involving a minimum of 25 repetitions per day, with three to four times that number being better, would seem an appropriate prescription. Most of this practice can be done at home, but the clinician would do well to see the patient at least once weekly to guarantee that progress is occurring and make appropriate refinements. Because of a lack of systematically increasing resistance, strengthening is unlikely.

The Evidence

Using computed tomography (CT), Hirano et al. (1999) reported increased closure at the level of the glottis and laryngeal entrance when using this technique. The study population included a small group of participants—5 healthy subjects and 3 subjects status-post surgical treatment for oral cancer. No data exist for movement disorders. Presumably the method could be expected to have an influence similar to the hard swallow (see below).

HARD (EFFORTFUL) SWALLOW

Description of Method

In its simplest form, this treatment requires only that the patient be instructed to swallow as hard or with as much effort as possible. Its apparent simplicity may be misleading, however. Clinicians would do well to demonstrate what is meant and then carefully monitor patient performance. Using the last part of the Showa instruction, which is to "contract all the muscles in your face, mouth, and neck," would seem to be a useful part of the instructions. This technique was introduced by Kahrilas and colleagues in a series of papers (1991, 1992a, 1992b, 1993).

Modifications

Other descriptions of how the method is to be executed are:

1. Logemann (1998) provides instruction for the patient to effortfully squeeze with all the tongue and throat muscles.
2. Another possibility is to squeeze the tongue and elevate the larynx as high as possible, and then swallow (Pouderoux & Kahrilas, 1995).
3. One modification in the case of significant velopharyngeal incompetence (VPI) is that the method may need to be softened or avoided altogether.
4. Most modifications lead one to the Showa maneuver, which is a more generalized and perhaps more general treatment and therefore a better alternative in most instances, as has already been described.

Effect

As with the Showa, the effects of the hard swallow on swallowing performance may be:

1. Enhanced posterior tongue movement and thereby closer approximation of the tongue back and posterior pharyngeal wall
2. More forceful propulsion of the bolus into and through the pharynx
3. Reduced oral residue
4. Reduced vallecular residue
5. Perhaps overall better timing of the onset of other pharyngeal components of the swallow
6. Possibly fewer penetration and aspiration events

The mechanism for these changes may be the placebo effect and increased neural activation. As resistance is not systematically manipulated, increased strength is unlikely, although endurance might be increased. As with the Showa, it may build skill, in which case nervous system change in the neural support of the swallow may occur as skill improves. As such, permanent effects after the method is ended cannot be expected. With practice, however, successful performance may require less conscious evocation of enhanced neural activation, assuming this is one mechanism of change.

Frequency and Duration

General principles apply. If the aim is to achieve a placebo effect and increase neural drive, then a few (perhaps as few as three) closely spaced sessions may be sufficient. If skill training is the goal, then intensive practice for a minimum of 6 weeks at a frequency of 6 out of 7 days, involving a minimum of 25 repetitions per day, with three to four times that number being better, would seem appropriate.

Again, much of this practice can be done at home, but we advise at least weekly clinic visits to guarantee that increased skill in its performance is occurring. If increased endurance is the goal, then the same schedule as for skill development is appropriate, with the exception that increasing the number of repetitions up to 100 repetitions of the exercise per day would appear sensible.

Candidacy

The following signs would seem to prompt use of this method:

1. Inadequate posterior-superior movement of the tongue when initiating the swallow
2. Slow, inadequate movement of the bolus through the pharynx and into the UES
3. Large pharyngeal residuals, perhaps especially in the valleculae
4. Perhaps reduced duration and extent of UES opening during the swallow
5. Inability to perform the Showa for motor or cognitive reasons
6. Presumed or documented pharyngeal weakness that cannot be strengthened, in which case greater force of lingual propulsion may be a partial compensation
7. Swallows that are incoordinated or impaired by reduced endurance
8. Aspiration or penetration due to decreased laryngeal closure

One contraindication is significant VPI.

The Evidence

We could not discover any studies of the hard swallow in those with movement disorders. Huckabee and Pelletier reported in 1999 that "the effect of this treatment is not well documented." Ten years later, the data are still sparse. Bulow and colleagues (2001, 2002) studied the effortful swallow in eight patients with stroke and head and neck cancer and found reduced depth of penetration, but no change in the number of misdirected swallows or peak amplitude or duration of intrabolus pressure. Lazarus and colleagues (2002) found the effortful swallow increased tongue base and pharyngeal pressures and duration of contact in three patients with head and neck cancer. In a larger group of healthy participants, Hind et al. (2001) found that the effortful swallow increased oral pressures and amount of oral residue as well as a number of durational measures (anterior hyolaryngeal movement, laryngeal closure, and UES opening).

INTENTION/ATTENTION TREATMENTS

Description of Methods

Intention/attention treatments are only now being introduced into treatment of the panoply of motor disorders, including swallowing. As a result, no formal protocols have been created. In the interest of making clinicians aware of emerging trends, however, some general treatment procedures are included here. Clinicians are reminded that these treatments are new and their effects merely speculative.

Intention may be improved by having the patient capable of feeding herself initiate the swallow by making a large sweeping arm and hand gesture while bringing the utensil full of food up to the mouth. In other words, the patient would load the fork and then perform a grand sweeping gesture with the utensil as it approaches the mouth. In this instance, the patient is urged to swallow quickly upon the food's being placed in the mouth. The exception, of course, is for food that must be chewed first.

An alternative is for the patient to be taught to make a pointing gesture or touch a dot or other target in either right or left hemispace with either the right or left hand immediately prior to initiating the swallow. In this instance, the bolus would be in the mouth and prepared for swallowing prior to the gesture.

Placing food and drink in either right or left hemispace or having the patient direct attention to it may influence attentional mechanisms and be associated with improved eating or swallowing.

Modifications

Most of what gets done in these new and essentially untested approaches qualifies as modification in the absence of a coherent, data-based protocol. Here are a few modifications of the basic approaches above that we have tried:

1. The clinician supports the arm and guides it in an arc if the patient is having difficulty.
2. Have the patient imitate the clinician if she is having difficulty.
3. Have the patient touch a colored spot or other target, even one that lights up or makes a sound, if pointing does not work.
4. The clinician can establish a treatment routine in which the patient is taught to swallow immediately after the clinician completes whatever act is selected from above.
5. Cues can be faded.

6. In the future, vibrating, noise-making, and illuminated utensils and dishes may be used to influence attention.

Effects

If these approaches are to influence eating and swallowing, those influences will be obvious within one or two sessions. One might expect increased eating and quicker swallowing, with less time spent manipulating or holding individual boluses. The placebo and increased neural activation effects are the most likely explanations.

Candidacy

These methods may be promising for movement disorders patients who eat slowly, inadequately, or variably and who are recognizable because food remains on the plate or in their mouths for inordinate periods of time. It can be hypothesized that in the absence of sensory abnormalities such as field cuts or profound weakness or illness, these signs may well result from intention/attention deficits, in which case candidacy can be defined as:

1. Having difficulty with initiation of movements
2. Having difficulty with sustaining attention

Frequency and Duration

Patients for whom these methods may be appropriate are likely to have severe illness and a variety of cognitive impairments. Therefore, it can be hypothesized that treatment will need to be frequent, especially in the first 1 or 2 weeks. Caregivers will need to provide more or less constant cueing. Patient independence is unlikely. Independence, if it does come, will be unlikely before 6 to 8 weeks of daily practice

The Evidence

No data have ever been published to our knowledge.

NEUROMUSCULAR ELECTRICAL STIMULATION (NMES)

The Methods

Electrical stimulation alone or as a precursor to a swallow attempt has been administered to three body sites in a variety of patients. Those three sites are: (a) the exterior neck over the suprahyoid musculature, (b) the faucial pillars (Power et al., 2004, 2006), and (c) the posterior pharyngeal wall (Fraser et al., 2002). A variety of frequencies and durations of electrical stimulation have been reported. *These treatments require specialized training, and this book is not the appropriate venue for this training.* However, the outline of a variety of methodologies will be presented. The interested reader will want to seek out specialized training and further explore the literature.

External application of electrical stimulation to the muscles of the neck has been accomplished with a variety of stim-

ulator arrays. Common sites are bilaterally on the suprahyoid musculature, multiple sites at the midline of this musculature, and bilaterally over the suprahyoids and larynx. Larsen (1973) was perhaps the first to describe this approach. He reported a brief period of electrical stimulation delivered to the larynx at the level of the thyroid notch resulted in the elevation of the larynx and the appearance of a swallow. More recently, a number of authors have reported the benefit of variations of this approach, typically combined with a variety of traditional swallowing treatments (Blumenfeld, Hahn, Lepage, Leonard, & Belafsky, 2006; Leelamanit, Limsakul, & Geater, 2002; Shaw et al., 2007).

Power and colleagues (2004, 2006) have reported experimental findings on the application of electrical stimulation to the faucial pillars accomplished using a digitally applied electrode. In their first study using healthy adults, high-frequency stimulation (5 Hz) was found to produce cortical inhibition and decreased swallow function during videofluoroscopy. Contrastingly, low-frequency stimulation (0.2 Hz) produced increased cortical excitability, which did not influence normal swallowing (Power et al., 2004). In follow-up work in a group of 16 stroke patients with dysphagia, low-frequency stimulation (0.2 Hz) or sham stimulation was again delivered to the faucial pillars. No effect was found in either treatment group on temporal measures of swallowing or PAS score 60 minutes after stimulation. The authors suggested that additional work is required to determine "optimal stimulation parameters and timing of any potential beneficial effect" (Power et al., 2006, p. 54)

Stimulation of the posterior pharyngeal wall has been accomplished with a single electrode located against the posterior pharyngeal wall at approximately the mid cervical spine (Fraser et al., 2002). In healthy participants, researchers found that electrical stimulation could either facilitate or inhibit corticobulbar excitability, depending on the parameters of stimulation delivered. For example, 1 or 5 Hz stimulation increased corticobulbar excitability, whereas 10, 20, and 40 Hz stimulation had the opposite effect. The optimal stimulation parameters with healthy participants were found to be 5 Hz stimulation at 75% of maximum tolerated intensity for 10 minutes. These parameters of stimulation were then applied to acute stroke patients with dysphagia, which resulted in increases in corticobulbar excitability that correlated with improvements in swallowing (based on VFSE) for at least 60 minutes after stimulation.

Modifications

Stimulation of the external neck admits to a variety of site, order, frequency, intensity, and duration modifications accompanied or unaccompanied by a swallow after every stimulation. Many more data are needed to understand the effect of these variables on the swallow and to determine the optimal parameters of stimulation.

Shorter periods of stimulation each followed by a swallow and bilateral stimulation are logical modifications of the faucial pillar stimulation described above.

Similarly, shorter periods of stimulation and a swallow subsequent to each is a logical modification of the pharyngeal stimulation. Presumably, sites higher and lower in the pharynx might also warrant investigation.

Effects

The possibility of a placebo effect is high, given the high-tech appearance of this approach. Freed and colleagues (2001) hypothesize an increase in tone "to the point where exercise may strengthen or activate the muscle" (p. 472). They also mention the possibility of facilitating the swallow reflex. Because electrical stimulation has been used longer and studied more carefully in physical therapy, the literature on effects for the extremities is somewhat clearer. Reducing atrophy and increasing strength and endurance have been reported (Stein et al., 2002), for example, especially when stimulation is combined with resistance training. It is possible that these improvements could support further skill development as well.

Frequency and Duration

Crary and colleagues (2007) report survey results on frequency and duration of treatment. Three 1-hour sessions per week or five 1-hour sessions per week were the most common patterns of practice. Duration of treatment was most likely to be between 11 and 20 treatment sessions.

Candidacy

Based on the same report by Crary and colleagues (2007), the usual population for stimulation would appear to be stroke, and the sign that most frequently causes clinicians to consider the method is aspiration. Freed and colleagues (2001) enrolled any patient with evidence of dysphagia on instrumental examination.

The implication, apparently, is of a systemic effect of electrical stimulation on the swallowing mechanism.

The Evidence

Carnaby-Mann and Crary (2007) performed a meta-analysis to further determine the effect of transcutaneous electrical stimulation on swallowing rehabilitation. Based on seven studies that met inclusion criteria, "a small but significant summary effect size" was found (Carnaby-Mann & Crary, 2007, p. 564). Improvements in swallowing as evidenced by oral diet advancement and reduced aspiration were the most frequently reported outcomes of the clinicians surveyed by Crary and colleagues (2007). Importantly, no treatment-related adverse events were reported by respondents.

TACTILE-THERMAL APPLICATION

Description of the Method

Tactile-thermal application (TTA) is performed using frozen ice sticks, which are rubbed against the faucial pillars and sides of tongue bilaterally prior to providing directions to the patient to swallow. Specifically, the steps are as follows:

1. Ice sticks are frozen.
2. Once frozen, they are plunged in ice to keep them frozen while being used one at a time.
3. The patient is instructed about the procedures.
4. An ice stick is withdrawn from the ice, the patient is instructed to open her mouth, and the clinician gently and systematically introduces the ice stick and moves it toward the faucial pillars.
5. When the faucial pillars are contacted, the clinician provides three swipes of the ice stick against the pillars and sides of tongue, beginning from as inferior as possible, first on one side and then on the other.
6. The ice stick is withdrawn and the patient is instructed to swallow.
7. Sequence is repeated beginning with the pillars on the opposite side.
8. After every trial, the clinician asks about feelings of cold and of comfort.

Modifications

Modifications may include:

1. Use a chilled laryngeal mirror if the patient has an unacceptable amount of aspiration of the water created by the melting ice stick.
2. Begin stimulation farther forward in the mouth and systematically desensitize a gag or other extreme response that might occur by beginning at the faucial pillars.
3. Use flavored ice sticks (sweet or sour) if greater taste seems appropriate.
4. Increase duration between trials if uncomfortable.
5. Reduce number of strokes on each side if uncomfortable.
6. Abandon cold and use only touch and movement if discomfort seems related to temperature.
7. Encourage more than one swallow —up to five—after each administration of stimulation.
8. Supply additional bolus (water from the melting ice will accumulate in the

mouth) immediately after stimulation and before urging the patient to swallow.

9. Instruct the patient to hard swallow after stimulation.

Frequency and Duration

These variables have not been established in movement disorders. In stroke, minimum frequency and duration are:

1. Sixty to 90 trials per day.
2. Absolute minimum of 4 weeks.
3. Absolute minimum of 5 days per week.
4. More of all three is probably better.

Effects

The physiologic effects of TTA are based solely on speculation. One hypothesis is that TTA lowers the threshold for effective initiation of the swallow. Behaviorally, the effects may include increased responsiveness of the pharyngeal swallowing response and improved airway protection if penetration and aspiration events are related to delayed initiation of the swallow.

Candidacy

Candidates are patients with slow swallow initiation resulting in penetration or aspiration or slow swallow initiation with functional consequences, such as unacceptably long times to finish a meal.

Slow responses are not necessarily bad responses in need of treatment. Therefore, this method is contraindicated if:

1. Slowness has no functional consequences, such as unacceptably slow eating.
2. Slowness is not accompanied by penetration or aspiration or convincing evidence that these events are more likely to occur at slower as opposed to faster rates.

The Evidence

Rosenbek and colleagues (Rosenbek, Robbins, Fishback, & Levine, 1991; Rosenbek, Roecker, Wood, & Robbins, 1996; Rosenbek et al., 1998) have systematically studied the effects of TTA in stroke patients with dysphagia. The data suggest that TTA may shorten total swallow duration and initiation of the swallow in some patients.

OTHER POSTERIOR TONGUE MANEUVERS

Description of Methods

A variety of exercises posited to enhance posterior tongue to posterior pharyngeal wall movement have been described. The four discussed below are the: hawk maneuver, gargling, feigned yawn, and forcible posterior tongue retraction. The goal of all four is to enhance posterior tongue motion. The danger with these activities as with all such so-called oral motor exercises is their failure to satisfy the principle of specificity. Another danger, albeit not one with the methods but with their application, is that such exercises are often provided with little physiologic rationale (see Candidacy) and measurement of either their adequacy during practice or their treatment effects. Hence, they are added here with some trepidation and with the caveat that doing nothing may be no worse than their inappropriate use.

Hawk Maneuver

The activity's purpose is described. Patients are reminded that the goal is not to say *hawk* or any other word ending in /k^/, but to use the word to enhance posterior tongue valving for the swallow. Therefore, a bit of description of the tongue's activity and importance to swallowing is usually necessary. Also, it is to be emphasized that normal sounding /k^/ is not the goal. Indeed, it should be abnormally forceful and explosive.

The patient is instructed to say the word *hawk* with exaggerated posterior tongue placement and force. The patient practices and the clinician provides KR as appropriate. Repeat. Begin the swallowing exercise with or without a bolus with instruction to the patient to achieve the same exaggerated, forced tongue movement to initiate the swallow.

Gargling

This activity's purpose is described. The emphasis is on control of the posterior tongue. The patient is instructed to take a small sip of some satisfying liquid and then gargle it. Gargling is difficult to teach, although the clinician can demonstrate. Generally, if this action is not more or less automatic, the method should be abandoned. Repeat. Have the patient begin swallowing using the same exaggerated, forced tongue movement to initiate the swallow.

Yawn

This activity's purpose is described. The clinician should demonstrate as realistic a yawn as possible and have the patient imitate. It is important for the patient to emphasize exaggerated superior and posterior tongue movement. The yawn will potentially not be as useful if the tongue is merely moved posteriorly. Repeat. Have the patient begin swallowing using the same exaggerated, forced tongue movement to initiate the swallow.

Forcible Posterior Tongue Retraction

The activity's purpose is described. The clinician demonstrates. The patient tries to duplicate exaggerated, forced tongue elevation and retraction. Repeat. Have the patient begin swallowing using the same exaggerated movement to initiate the swallow.

Modifications

Modifications on such superficially simple procedures are few, assuming patient understanding and clinician diligence. Of course, the patient can be given other words ending in /k^/ for variety during the hawk maneuver. A bolus can be deleted on the gargle if the patient aspirates significantly, though without a bolus this exercise is even harder and is likely to be unsuccessful. Imaging may enhance the yawn and even the posterior tongue movement. It is impossible to exaggerate how important it is to try transferring any of these movements to swallowing.

Effects

Even a few sessions of these activities may create a placebo effect and enhance neural activation. They will not improve skill unless systematically carried over from the exercise to tongue movement during swallow. Strengthening should not be expected, but multiple repetitions may improve endurance. Behaviorally, the effect may be enhanced tongue-pharyngeal wall approximation upon the initiation of the swallow.

Frequency and Duration

Minimum practice guidelines based on our clinical experience are 50 to 100 repetitions per day, 6 days per week, for a minimum of 6 weeks. If successful, then a regimen of 100 repetitions per day, 3 days per week for maintenance may suffice.

Candidacy

Candidates include those with poor posterior tongue to pharyngeal wall approximation.

The Evidence

Limited data are available. Veis, Logemann, and Colangelo (2000) studied posterior tongue retraction in 20 consecutive patients referred for VFSE during pudding swallows, forcible tongue retraction, yawn, and gargle tasks. Gargle resulted in the most tongue base retraction.

15 Parkinson's Disease

This chapter, like all the disease chapters, is organized for easy review. It begins with definitions, followed by general signs and symptoms, epidemiology, evaluation, and treatment. Swallowing is featured in the second, longer section.

DEFINITION

Parkinson's disease (PD) is a chronic progressive neurodegenerative disease that begins in the brainstem and progresses to involve the entire brain (Braak, Ghebremedhin, Rub, Bratzke, & Del Tredici, 2004; Braak et al., 2003; Braak et al., 2006). However, the cardinal manifestations of bradykinesia/hypokinesia, rigidity, tremor, and postural instability are thought to be predominantly attributable to basal ganglia disease, including reduction of dopamine in the striatum, particularly the putamen (Bergman & Deuschl, 2002). PD is common, particularly in the elderly. In fact, among neurodegenerative conditions, only Alzheimer's disease is encountered more frequently (Nussbaum & Ellis, 2003). The cause of PD is unknown, but genetic and environmental influences (and their interactions) are thought to be involved. Most cases of PD occur sporadically, though a relatively small proportion of cases appear to be inherited.

SIGNS/DIAGNOSTIC CRITERIA

Main signs are: (a) bradykinesia/hypokinesia, (b) rigidity, (c) tremor, and (d) postural instability. *Bradykinesia/hypokinesia* refers to slowness in the onset and execution of volitional and nonvolitional movements, as well as a poverty of the amount and quality of movement. Behaviorally, these movement abnormalities may result in decreased arm swing with walking, *masked facies* (or *hypomimia*), and a shuffling, hesitant gait. Muscle *rigidity* occurs when the resistance of a joint to passive movement is increased. Patients will often describe a sensation of stiffness or an inability to relax their limb muscles. *Tremor* is often the most conspicuous sign of PD. Most typically, PD is associated with a resting tremor with a frequency of 4–7 Hz (Klockgether, 2004). Clinical criteria for diagnosis of PD usually include the presence of bradykinesia/hypokinesia with rigidity and/or tremor. In addition to the classic triad of PD signs is often added a fourth —*postural instability*. This sign is tested with the pull test, in which the clinician stands behind the patient and pulls back on his shoulders. Patients with postural instability will demonstrate a decreased ability to correct their posture and may even fall if left unsupported. Symptoms of this sign reported by patients include falls, unsteadiness, and poor balance. Signs are generally unilateral upon onset, and although bilateral involvement is expected with disease progression, an asymmetry may persist (Fernandez, Rodriguez, Skidmore, & Okun, 2007). The possibility that the onset of right-sided signs is associated with earlier, more severe swallowing problems has been posited but not demonstrated experimentally.

The usual measure of sign severity in PD is the Unified Parkinson's Disease Rating Scale (UPDRS; Fahn, Elton, & UPDRS program members, 1987). Table 15–1 summarizes the various components of this measure. A lower score indicates less severe disease. The UPDRS is often administered in the on and off medication conditions as a measure of treatment benefit.

The Activities of Daily Living portion of the UPDRS includes items concerning both salivation and swallowing. Scoring is accomplished with a five-point rating scale. As can be seen in Table 15–2, only a gross estimate of the patient's performance is provided.

EVOLUTION OVER TIME

Signs worsen and bilateral involvement develops over time, though asymmetry may persist. Increasing falls; decline in ability to complete activities of daily living; a festinating gait; *micrographia*; an increasingly severe speech deficit, called *hypokinetic dysarthria* and characterized by inadequate loudness, consonant imprecision, rate abnormalities, and decline in prosodic features; and cognitive decline can occur. Ultimately, the typical person with PD becomes nearly incapable of independent movement. Death is often the result of aspiration. A variety of scales are employed to quantify the disease's advance, including the UPDRS and the Hoehn and Yahr staging scale (Hoehn & Yahr, 1967) shown in Table 15–3. Modifications to the latter scale have been proposed, such as the use of 0.5 increments, but it has been suggested that the original five-point scale be maintained at the present time (Goetz et al., 2004).

EPIDEMIOLOGY

Onset is typically between ages 40 and 70, with the average age of diagnosis being 62 (de Rijk et al., 1997). Onset can occasionally occur in younger people. Men are more often affected than women and whites more frequently than African Americans and Asians, but it is present in

Table 15–1. Components of the Unified Parkinson's Disease Rating Scale (UPDRS)

Components of the UPDRS
Part I, Mentation, Behavior, and Mood
Part II, Activities of Daily Living
Part III, Motor Exam
Part IV, Complications

Note. From "The Unified Parkinson's Disease Rating Scale," by S. Fahn, R. L. Elton, and UPDRS program members, 1987, in S. Fahn, C. D. Marsden, D. B. Calne, and M. Goldstein (Eds.), *Recent Developments in Parkinson's Disease* (Vol. 2, pp. 153–163), Florham Park, NJ: Macmillan Healthcare Information. Reprinted with permission.

Table 15–2. Items 6 and 7 from the Unified Parkinson's Disease Rating Scale (UPDRS) on salivation and swallowing

Salivation Scale	Description
0	Normal
1	Slight but definite excess of saliva in mouth; may have nighttime drooling
2	Moderately excessive saliva; may have minimal drooling
3	Marked excess of saliva with some drooling
4	Marked drooling; requires constant tissue or handkerchief

Swallowing Scale	Description
0	Normal
1	Rare choking
2	Occasional choking
3	Requires soft food
4	Requires NG or gastrostomy feeding

Note. From "The Unified Parkinson's Disease Rating Scale," by S. Fahn, R. L. Elton, and UPDRS program members, 1987, in S. Fahn, C. D. Marsden, D. B. Calne, and M. Goldstein (Eds.), *Recent Developments in Parkinson's Disease* (Vol. 2, pp. 153–163), Florham Park, NJ: Macmillan Healthcare Information. Reprinted with permission.

Table 15–3. The Hoehn and Yahr Staging Scale

Stage	Description
Stage I	Unilateral involvement only, usually with minimal or no functional impairment.
Stage II	Bilateral or midline involvement, without impairment of balance.
Stage III	First sign of impaired righting reflexes. Functionally, the patient is somewhat restricted in his activities but may have some work potential, depending on the type of employment. Patients are physically capable of leading independent lives and their disability is mild to moderate.
Stage IV	Fully developed, severely disabling disease; the patient is able to walk and stand unassisted but is markedly incapacitated.
Stage V	Confinement to bed or wheelchair unless aided.

Note. From "Parkinsonism: Onset, Progression and Mortality," by M. M. Hoehn and M. D. Yahr, 1967, *Neurology*, 17, pp. 427–442. Reprinted by permission.

all countries. Prevalence is estimated to be 31 to 328 per 100,000 worldwide, and 1% to 2% of persons 65 or older have PD. In the United States, the cost of care for those with PD is estimated to be 26 billion dollars (Levine et al., 2003).

MEDICAL/SURGICAL MANAGEMENT

Medical treatments are preferred as first line treatments for PD, although they may be delayed until the signs of the condition have a functional impact. Often a single drug and then combinations of drugs are systematically introduced in the search for an effective treatment or as a single medication loses its effectiveness. Once reasonable drug trials confirm that medications alone are not as effective as the patient, family, and medical team want them to be, surgical treatments may be considered.

Medical Management

A number of medications may be employed in the treatment of PD. What follows is a listing of pharmacological agents that may be encountered. For further details on this complicated and rapidly expanding subject, see Stacy (2000) and Horstink and colleagues (2006a, 2006b).

1. Carbidopa/levodopa
2. Dopamine agonists (e.g., pergolide, pramipexole, ropinirole)
3. Anticholinergics (e.g., benztropine, trihexyphenidyl)
4. Amantadine
5. COMT inhibitors (e.g., tolcapone, entacapone)

6. MAO-B inhibitors (e.g., selegiline, rasagiline)

Surgical Management

Surgical management of PD is usually only considered in patients with disabling motor symptoms that are insufficiently controlled with medical management. Although surgical management of PD was largely discontinued with the introduction of levodopa in 1967 and its widespread use by the 1970s, interest in this area had been renewed over the last two decades.

Surgical Ablation

The use of lesion therapy in PD (and other movement disorders) has a long history. Although it has been replaced at many centers by deep brain stimulation (DBS; see below), lesion surgery for PD may still be encountered. The primary ablative procedures and their surgical targets are as follows:

1. Thalamotomy typically involves lesion of the ventralis intermedius nucleus (VIM) of the thalamus.
2. Pallidotomy most commonly targets the globus pallidus pars interna (GPi) of the basal ganglia.
3. Subthalamotomy is the least commonly encountered ablative surgery for PD. The surgical target is the subthalamic nucleus (STN) of the basal ganglia.

Deep Brain Stimulation

DBS is a surgical procedure in which electrical stimulation is delivered through chronically implanted electrodes to treat the motor signs of PD. DBS is most commonly applied to the following neural targets in PD:

1. VIM
2. GPi
3. STN

Complications

No curative treatments are currently available for PD; consequently, disease progression is inevitable in this neurodegenerative condition. In addition, as with all medical/surgical treatments, complications or adverse side effects are possible, including the following.

Complications of Medical Management

Dyskinesias are relatively quick hyperkinetic movements associated with prolonged levodopa therapy. These may occur in any body part including the head, mouth, tongue, and pharynx.

Dystonia is a pattern of abnormal muscle contraction causing abnormal posturing of any body structure including those involved in swallowing. Dystonia may be induced by levodopa during "wearing off" (see below) or when levodopa levels are rising or falling.

Wearing off occurs when the benefit of levodopa is decreased between doses. Medication benefit is typically predictable early in the disease, but with disease progression, wearing off may occur unpredictably or suddenly.

"Off" period dystonia may occur between dosages or early in the morning. *"On-off" fluctuations* are unpredictable and, at times, sudden changes in an individual's response to medicaton. *Dose failure* occurs when a lack of benefit occurs after medication ingestion.

Complications of Surgical Treatment

Surgical treatment of PD, particularly using DBS, is expensive and requires frequent follow-up for programming the device. Both ablative techniques and DBS may result in serious adverse events such as hemorrhage, stroke, infection, and subdural hematoma. Cognitive decline following surgery may occur. Speech decline may also occur following surgery, particularly following bilateral procedures.

Influence on Swallowing

Influence of medical and surgical management of PD on swallowing cannot be predicted but instead must be measured. However, in most cases, swallowing is not improved by medical/surgical management and may be associated with dysphagia. In particular, when surgery is performed bilaterally, the onset of dysphagia or an increase in its severity may be encountered.

SWALLOWING IN PD

Epidemiology

Depending on how sensitively dysphagia is measured, swallowing abnormalities occur in nearly 100% of men and women with PD some time in the disease's course, being more frequent as disease severity increases and potentially as surgical managements are added to medical ones. For most patients, medications appear to have a neutral effect on swallowing. However, recent research from Lim et al. (2008) suggests that swallowing efficiency may be reduced with levodopa, although no effect on penetration or aspiration was found. In our experience, as side effects such as dyskinesia from prolonged levodopa exposure occur, swallowing may decline. Swallowing is seldom improved by ablative surgery or DBS, and even when performed with extreme competence, swallowing (and speech) may be negatively affected. Often, the health care team, family, and patient must decide which side effects are a reasonable trade-off for improved control of tremor and other motor signs of PD. Abnormalities can be expected in all phases of the swallow, including the esophageal stage. Be prepared, however, for patients to minimize or ignore symptoms (Bushmann, Dobmeyer, Leeker, & Perlmutter, 1989).

Symptoms

When patients do recognize and report symptoms, one of the earliest they report is difficulty swallowing pills. They frequently report pills sticking at a point they identify as high in the neck (at or just below the level of the larynx) or under the sternum. The full range of symptoms of both swallowing and eating abnormalities is also possible, even as first signs. These may be reported by patient or caregiver, and the clinician must be careful to differentiate symptoms caused by limb movement abnormality, which may make preparing and moving food and drink to the mouth difficult, from symptoms related to the swallowing structures. Symptoms include the following.

1. Coughing or choking on food and liquid
2. Excess saliva, although Ertekin (2002) suggests saliva flow remains constant but the number of saliva swallows is reduced

3. Choking or coughing on saliva
4. Drooling
5. Food falling from mouth
6. Food and liquid sticking in mouth or throat
7. Thick mucus
8. Difficulty chewing
9. Impaired taste and smell
10. Loss of appetite
11. Weight loss
12. Increased length of time required for meals

Signs

The following list of signs is derived primarily from videofluoroscopic swallow examinations, because this procedure has been most frequently used in studies of swallowing in those with PD. They are divided into oral, pharyngeal, and laryngeal signs. The reader is again cautioned that these stages are to a large degree arbitrary and that an abnormality in one can result from abnormalities in any of the others. Even oral stage abnormalities may result from a patient's fear that he will choke rather than from any primary oral phase deficit.

Oral Stage

Signs in the oral stage include:

1. Rocking movement of the bolus
2. Slowness to initiate oral manipulation
3. Slowness in anterior to posterior movement of the bolus to initiate the rest of the swallowing sequence
4. Failure to confine the bolus at the front of the mouth (i.e., drooling)
5. Failure to confine the bolus at the back of the mouth (i.e., premature spillage)

6. Impaired ability to prepare solid bolus efficiently
7. Oral residue after the swallow

Pharyngeal Stage

In our experience, pharyngeal stage signs can be highly variable but may include the following:

1. Bolus may move abnormally slowly or rapidly through the pharynx and upper esophageal sphincter (UES).
2. UES opening may be abnormally short and extent of opening may be reduced.
3. Upward and forward motion of the hyoid may be reduced.
4. Material enters the pharynx to the level of valleculae or pyriform sinuses prior to initiation of pharyngeal stage swallow (i.e., pharyngeal swallow delay).
5. Postswallow residue in the valleculae or pyriform sinuses, and on the aryepiglottic folds or posterior pharyngeal wall, may occur.
6. Residue of solids in the valleculae occurs frequently.
7. Reduced velopharyngeal competence for swallowing is *infrequent*, and if it occurs, an alternative diagnosis should be considered.
8. Pharyngeal stage function is often less severely involved than the oral stage until late in the disease.

Larynx

Activity of the larynx is usually included with a description of the pharyngeal stage. We separate it so as to be able to feature penetration and aspiration events.

1. Penetration above or to the level of the vocal folds is common, especially for liquids.

2. Often, the patient fails to react to this penetration.
3. Aspiration is infrequent until the disease progresses to an advanced stage.
4. Aspiration may occur more frequently in those with abnormally rapid pharyngeal movements.
5. Inadequate laryngeal closure during the swallow is increasingly frequent as disease progresses.
6. Silent aspiration may occur but is infrequent in our experience until very late in the disease's course.

Functional/QOL Influences

In our experience, perceived QOL impact of dysphagia is generally less in PD than in some other populations. Nonetheless, a variety of functional and psychological consequences are reported:

1. Slowness of eating, requiring increased length of time for meals
2. "Messy eating" for a variety of reasons
3. Reluctance to eat in public also for a variety of reasons
4. Embarrassment about drooling of saliva, food, and drink
5. Fear of choking
6. Having to leave the table to try to dislodge food at the sink

Health Consequences

Dysphagia can have serious health consequences for men and women with PD. Aspiration pneumonia, for example, is one of the leading causes of death in this population. The following health consequences need to be considered when planning treatment for PD patients:

1. Aspiration pneumonia
2. Weight loss

3. Dehydration
4. Anorexia
5. Disturbed sleep

Swallowing Evaluation

The procedures for the history, clinical swallow examination (CSE), videofluoroscopic swallow examination (VFSE), and the endoscopic swallow examination appear in Chapters 4–7. The emphasis here is only on the special observations and procedure modifications that might be critical to the best evaluation in PD.

Chart Review and History

Do not neglect a thorough history. Its results will help focus subsequent examinations and provide potentially crucial information to treatment planning. All questions from the history (see Chapter 4) can be employed, and in addition, the following may be of assistance.

1. Relationship of symptoms to medication schedule
2. Relationships between protein consumption and medication effects that might influence dietary recommendations
3. Other patterns in swallowing difficulty such as time of day, type of food and drink, posture, and so on
4. Sensory change, specifically in taste and smell
5. Sleep patterns
6. Appetite
7. Influence of upper extremity control on eating
8. Fatigue/energy
9. Apathy/interest
10. Rate of eating and any other idiosyncratic behaviors such as gorging

Clinical Swallow Examination (CSE)

The CSE has an important role in PD evaluation, where the reason for eating/swallowing complaints may be multiple or otherwise complex. The Mini-Mental status examination (Folstein, Folstein, & McHugh, 1975), the Apathy Evaluation Scale (AES; Marin, Biedrzycki, & Firinciogullari, 1991—see Appendix C), and the SWAL-QOL (see Chapter 4 and Appendix A) are all informative to treatment planning and prognostication. All parts of the bulbar sensory-motor exam (see Chapter 5) can be administered.

The eating examination should also be completed when appropriate. Areas of particular attention include the following:

1. Recognition of and reaction to food and liquid
2. Ability to handle utensils and glassware
3. Pace of eating
4. Bolus sizes and sequencing of liquids and solids
5. Adequacy of dentures, if worn
6. Influence of distraction
7. Appreciation of food and drink
8. Posture during mealtime
9. Influence of any postural modifications
10. Changes in physical or mental status during the period of exam

Videofluoroscopic Swallow Examination (VFSE)

In general, the VFSE needs to be challenging if it is to provide information helpful to decision making. If possible, schedule the examination during the part of the patient's medicine cycle corresponding to patient's mealtime. If possible, approximate the patient's eating posture during the examination.

Compare swallowing with an improved posture, if possible. Include self-administered, large thin liquid and solid boluses, including bites of favorite foods, if possible. If safe, let the patient control liquid bolus size and rate during sequential swallows. If possible, combine oropharyngeal and esophageal examinations in whatever sequence is the standard in the facility.

When reading the film, attend to:

1. Oral stage abnormalities
2. Their influence on subsequent stage performance
3. Influence of the various durations on safety and adequacy of bolus movement

Videoendoscopic Swallow Examination

We generally select VFSE when an instrumental assessment of oropharyngeal swallowing is indicated due to the prominent oral stage dysphagia in individuals with PD. However, indications for use of videoendoscopy include:

1. Difficulty with secretion management. In contrast to VFSE, the videoendoscopic exam allows for direct visualization of pharyngeal/laryngeal secretions.
2. Fatigue/decreased swallowing performance as meals progress. Time is often limited during VFSE, and the videoendoscopic exam may be better suited for instrumental assessment of dysphagia when swallowing performance over a longer period of time is needed to determine the effect of fatigue.
3. Assessment of laryngeal integrity, particularly to evaluate for vocal fold bowing.

Behavioral Management

For maximum effect, the management of persons with PD should be team treatment. Swallowing is likely to be influenced by the timing and effect of medical/surgical treatments and by the physical, psychological, and intellectual consequences of PD as it advances. Therefore, decisions about swallowing procedures must be integrated into a total plan of care unless, of course, a clinician is seeing a person with PD who is not receiving any other management and if that additional management cannot be arranged. The importance of the speech-language pathologist (SLP) in swallow management cannot be exaggerated, as aspiration consequences are a frequent cause of death in PD. Treatment decisions will be influenced as well by the duration of illness. As the disease progresses, rehabilitative efforts may be of limited usefulness. However, early in the disease's course, aggressive rehabilitation is important, not only to improve swallowing efficiency, safety, and adequacy, but perhaps to provide a neuroprotective effect as well. The neuroprotective effects of exercise can only be hypothesized at present, of course. What follows is a list of general guidelines for treatment followed by recommendations for rehabilitative and compensatory approaches. General principles for dysphagia treatment in general as well as descriptions of specific treatments appear as separate chapters.

Compensatory Approaches

Recognize the interactions of some foods and beverages with PD medications when making dietary recommendations. For example, Gibbons (2000) suggests that dopaminergic medications be taken

30–60 minutes before meals because of possible interactions between amino acids in meats and dairy that can alter medication absorption.

Have patients and their families consider timing meals to the medicine cycle and to periods when the patient is most rested.

Recommend the safest, least invasive diet consistency, bolus size, eating rate, order of liquid and solid boluses, posture, and eating environment. Troche and colleagues (2008) investigated the effect of bolus consistency on timing and safety of swallow in 10 individuals with PD and found that thicker consistencies generally resulted in less penetration and aspiration than thinner consistencies. However, although dietary modifications may be necessary at times, particularly when other risk factors for pneumonia are present (see Chapter 4), such a decision should not be entered into lightly, and rehabilitation should always be considered.

Encourage support group attendance. Encourage general exercise, which need not be elaborate and may involve nothing more than being up for more hours than are spent sleeping. Encourage socialization.

Rehabilitative Techniques

The classification, principles, and procedures of rehabilitative techniques appear in Chapter 11 and Chapter 14. So as to reduce needless redundancy in each of the disorder chapters in this book, what follows is merely a listing of techniques with brief commentary. Readers will want to refer to the appropriate chapter for guidelines on performing each of these techniques.

Lee Silverman Voice Treatment (LSVT). One study from El Sharkawi and colleagues (2002) suggests that LSVT may influence oral and pharyngeal stage performance, particularly in terms of lingual biomechanics.

Expiratory Muscle Strength Training (EMST). The available data suggest that EMST may have a positive influence on swallowing (Wheeler, Chiara, & Sapienza, 2007), pulmonary function, and coughing (Kim & Sapienza, 2006).

Inspiratory Muscle Strength Training (IMST). Although data on the effects on swallowing are not yet available, this technique may be combined with EMST, and both may be combined with LSVT.

Other Techniques. Other techniques as described in Chapter 14 can be tried, of course, based on results of the swallowing exam(s).

SUMMARY

More is known about this condition's effect on swallowing than any other condition in this book. The critical message is that aggressive rehabilitation is justified.

16 Multiple System Atrophy

DEFINITION

The definition and therefore diagnosis of multiple system atrophy (MSA) is at least modestly controversial, although a set of criteria for its confident or probable diagnosis has been published by Gilman and colleagues (1999). It is one of the typical forms of atypical parkinsonism. According to Gilman et al. (1999), MSA is a "progressive neurodegenerative disease of unknown etiology [which] occurs sporadically and causes parkinsonism with cerebellar, autonomic, urinary, and pyramidal dysfunction in many combinations" (p. 94). This heterogeneous picture led Shulman and colleagues (2004) to create the diagram that appears in Figure 16–1. In this diagram, the Parkinson features are labeled as extrapyramidal, the autonomic as autonomic failure, and the cerebellar as idiopathic cerebellar ataxia. This diagram ignores the corticospinal deficits but is useful nonetheless. It allows the capture of older nomenclature represented as OPCA for *olivopontocerebellar atrophy*, SND for *striatonigral degeneration*, and SDS for *Shy-Drager syndrome*. Gilman and colleagues (1999), reporting on the results of a consensus conference charged with specifying the criteria for a diagnosis of MSA, urged retirement of this terminology. Regarding Shy-Drager

syndrome, Gilman et al. stated that it is "no longer useful" (p. 198) as a label for the patient with severe autonomic dysfunction. Instead, Gilman and his group recommend the nomenclature MSA-P and MSA-C, depending on whether parkinsonian or cerebellar features predominate. Because the older terms SND for MSA-P and OPCA for MSA-C persist, and because at least a modest literature has appeared especially about OPCA, these terms will continue to appear along with MSA-P and MSA-C in this chapter.

SIGNS AND DIAGNOSTIC CRITERIA

For a diagnosis of MSA-P (or SND) to be entertained, evidence of one or more of the following is required: tremor, postural instability, rigidity, and bradykinesia or slowness of movement. In MSA-P, response to anti-PD medications is absent or short-lived. For MSA-C (or OPCA) to be diagnosed, ataxia of gait, gaze-evoked *nystagmus*, ataxic dysarthria, and ataxia of the lower limbs should be present on clinical examination. Autonomic dysfunction, which can predominate or occur in combination with other signs, includes impotence, orthostatic hypotension, and

125

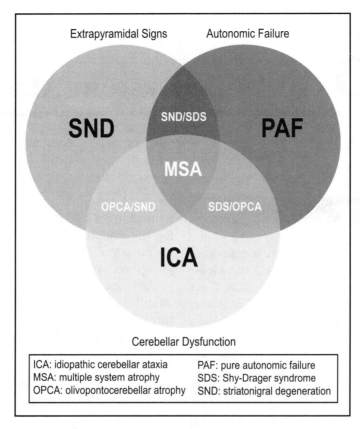

Figure 16–1. The relationship between multiple system atrophy (MSA) and related neurodegenerative conditions. *Note.* From "Multiple System Atrophy," by L. M. Shulman, A. Minagar, and W. J. Weiner, 2004, in R. L. Watts and W. C. Koller (Eds.), *Movement Disorders: Neurologic Principles and Practice* (2nd ed., pp. 359–369), New York: McGraw-Hill. Reprinted with permission.

urinary incontinence. Pyramidal involvement can also occur, sometimes even early in either condition's course and can include hyperreflexia, spasticity, and what Shulman and colleagues (2004) call *pseudobulbar palsy*. These same authors say that pyramidal signs can mask parkinsonian and cerebellar ones, as when spasticity slows movement and disguises ataxic incoordination. Table 16–1 from Gilman and colleagues (1999) shows criteria for possible, probable, and definite MSA (note that pyramidal signs do not figure in the diagnostic criteria).

EVOLUTION

MSA in all its forms is a progressive disorder. Onset is usually in the 50s, and death occurs within 1 to 18 years. Shul-

---

Table 16–1. Consensus criteria for diagnosis of possible, probable, and definite MSA

I. Possible MSA: one criterion plus two features from separate other domains. When the criterion is parkinsonism, a poor levodopa response qualifies as one feature (hence only one additional feature is required).

II. Probable MSA: criterion for autonomic failure/urinary dysfunction plus poorly levodopa responsive parkinsonism or cerebellar dysfunction.

III. Definite MSA: pathologically confirmed by the presence of a high density of glial cytoplasmic inclusions in association with a combination of degenerative changes in the nigrostriatal and olivopontocerebellar pathways.

Source: Gilman, Low, Quinn, Albanese, Ben-Shlomo, Fowler, et al., 1999. Republished with the permission of Elsevier.

---

man and colleagues (2004) report a median duration of disease of slightly more than 6 years.

EPIDEMIOLOGY

Men and women are equally likely to develop MSA. It is relatively rare, perhaps 0.6 cases for every 100,000 in the population (Vanacore et al., 2001). MSA-P is the most common manifestation in the West (Ben-Shlomo, Wenning, Tison, & Quinn, 1997). In Japan, MSA-C appears to be more common (Watanabe et al., 2002), and a high proportion of patients go on to develop parkinsonian, autonomic, and ataxic features.

MEDICAL/SURGICAL MANAGEMENT

Medical Management

Dopaminergic medications may have at least a short-term effect on signs in MSA in some patients, although response is quite variable and failure to respond to levodopa is considered diagnostic of MSA by some practitioners. Larger doses of medication and a shorter period of medical effectiveness may be the norm for persons who are dopa-responsive. Botulinum toxin injection in the case of dystonia as a further manifestation of MSA has been described. Thobois and colleagues (2001) report severe, persisting dysphagia following botulinum toxin for cervical dystonia requiring months of tube feeding in a lady with MSA.

Surgical Management

Deep brain stimulation (DBS) has been tried in individual cases, with generally unsatisfactory results. Santens and colleagues (2006), for example, implanted electrodes bilaterally in globus pallidus internus (GPi). The results were poor, with disabling akinesia leading to loss of mobility and more severe speech and swallowing problems. Interestingly, it was the left stimulator that appeared to account for the worsening of swallow. Tarsy and colleagues (2003) implanted bilateral subthalamic nucleus (STN) electrodes in one patient. General motor function improved, but swallowing declined. This approach was selected due to the patient's positive response to levodopa, though presumably this responsiveness did not extend to swallowing function. They advise against STN DBS in MSA.

Complications

The same side effects of medication reported in Parkinson's disease (PD) might be expected in the dopa-responsive patient with MSA.

Effects on Swallow

Thobois and colleagues (2001) report such a severe dysphagia following botulinum toxin injection for cervical dystonia that a patient had to have nasogastric feeding for 4 months. Santens et al.'s (2006) patient became so akinetic that initiation of the swallow was nearly impossible. Even turning the left stimulator "off" left the patient with severe oral stage abnormalities and what was described as "permanent problems with ingestion of liquids" (p. 182). The patient operated on by Tarsy and colleagues (2003) aspirated when the stimulators were on and did not when they were off.

SWALLOWING IN MSA

Epidemiology

Early discussions of MSA minimized the importance of dysphagia, though it is increasingly recognized. For example, Shulman and colleagues (2004) call it a "pervasive" sign, and Higo et al. (2005)

state that dysphagia "is the most critical complication of MSA" (p. 647). This notion is supported by data from Muller and colleagues (2001) who found a remaining survival time of 15 months after the onset of subjective complaint of dysphagia. Dysphagia, in rare cases, may be the presenting symptom (Berciano, 1982; Muller et al., 2001). Onset of dysphagia is likely to be earlier and more severe in MSA than in PD (Alfonsi et al., 2007; Wenning & Quinn, 1997).

Higo and colleagues (2003b) used VFSE to evaluate swallowing in 30 patients with MSA referred for swallowing assessment, and approximately 75% of patients exhibited at least one sign of dysphagia. Subjective complaint of dysphagia was present in 73% of the 15 patients with MSA studied by Muller and colleagues in 2001. Berciano (1982) reviewed a substantial literature on OPCA (which would now be called MSA-C by many) and describes dysphagia as a common sign. He computed a frequency of approximately one third and suggested that swallowing is most often impaired at the mid- and endpoints of the disease. Higo, Nito, and Tayama (2005) studied 29 patients with MSA-C referred for swallowing assessment with VFSE. They divided their patients into three groups based on the duration of disease. VFSE revealed at least one sign of dysphagia in about half of the subjects in the group only 1 to 3 years after disease onset. This increased to over 70% 7 years or more after onset. Dysphagia has been reported in 44% of patients identified with SND (or what many now call MSA-P) (Gouider-Khouja, Vidailhet, Bonnet, Pichon, & Agid, 1995).

Symptoms

Patients with MSA seem to recognize and admit their symptoms, perhaps to a greater degree than do those with PD (Sjostrom, Holmberg, & Strang, 2002). Eleven of 19 (58%) reported difficulty with swallowing, otherwise unspecified. One could predict that a partial listing would include drooling, choking, coughing, food sticking, food lodging in the mouth after the swallow, and increased length of meals.

Signs

Signs are increasingly well described. This discussion starts with laryngeal stridor. Stridor is not a sign of dysphagia but it is a sign of laryngeal involvement and, indeed, is often featured as one of the telltale signs of MSA-P.

Laryngeal stridor, which can be defined as the sound of obstructed breathing because of a narrowing of the airway at the level of the larynx, has been reported in 47% of a group of 36 MSA patients by Higo and colleagues (2003a). That group did not discover a significant relationship of stridor to dysphagia but did report stridor is more likely as the disease progresses. They warn against a tube-feeding decision being made solely on the basis of stridor. Whether stridor is the result of weakness or dystonia is debated, a debate that requires resolution because, if dystonic, botulinum toxin injection may be a treatment possibility (Merlo, Occhini, Pacchetti, & Alfonsi, 2002). The condition can advance to airway obstruction (Lim & Kennedy, 2007).

Oral Stage

Oral stage signs may be more severe than pharyngeal throughout the disease's course. Oral phrase difficulty, especially in lingual initiation of the swallow, appears to be very common. Higo and colleagues (2003b) identified it as the most common sign in 29 patients with MSA

(both MSA-P and MSA-C). They also identified reduced movement of the tongue base and "disturbance of bolus holding" (p. 632) as the next most significant signs. These signs increase in severity with duration of disease (Higo et al., 2005). Delayed oral activity of any sort with most boluses is a frequent sign in our clinical practice.

Pharyngeal Stage

Reduced hyolaryngeal movement is also common. Residuals in the pyriform sinuses and valleculae are often reported. UES hypertonicity may be present (Merlo et al, 2002; Alfonsi et al, 2007). This problem is more severe than in PD and can occur before the subjective complaint of dysphagia. This dysfunction is not necessarily predicted by disease duration or severity. It may be more common in MSA-C.

Laryngeal Stage

Aspiration is common as disease severity and duration increase. Pneumonia associated with aspiration may be a leading cause of death in this population.

Functional/Quality of Life Consequences

The forms of MSA are likely to be more aggressive than PD. Thus, swallowing impairment is likely to be more severe sooner and require more aggressive management. The impact on quality of life is therefore likely to be greater as well. Practitioners, teams, and the patient and family may well have to decide how aggressively to act. Altered diets may be tolerable if threats to pulmonary health are reduced. A decision about tube feeding in this illness, as in dementing illnesses, should not be made reflexively. With disease progression to a severe state, the prevention of aspiration will likely be impossible in many cases. An end to the socialization that can accompany shared meals can be harmful to life's quality. Of course, severe pulmonary complications can be as well. In general, modern practitioners justly yield to a patient's wishes or to those of a legal guardian, and a written plan for the end of life can make such decisions straightforward. As will be outlined below, our approach is to advocate for early and aggressive intervention and contributions to decisions that try to balance safety adequacy and pleasure.

Health Consequences

The threats to health of dysphagia are amply documented. Muller and colleagues (2001) established the predictive value of dysphagia on mortality in a variety of patient populations, including those with MSA. Specifically, they observed that "the latency to a complaint of dysphagia was highly correlated with total survival time" (p. 259). They reason that evaluation and treatment of dysphagia may prolong survival in this group. Higo and colleagues (2003b) found a history of aspiration pneumonia in 7 of their 29 patients, but with no correlation of pneumonia to aspiration on VFSE. Indeed, six of seven patients with a history of aspiration pneumonia did not aspirate on VFSE. The forms of MSA are usually relentless in their assault on the patient's health. Dysphagia contributes to the assault.

Evaluation

The principles and procedures of evaluation are presented in Chapters 4, 5, 6,

and 7. Here, we highlight special features that may be especially important in managing the dysphagia of MSA.

Chart Review and History

Because MSA patients can have variable mixes of parkinsonian, ataxic, autonomic, and pyramidal signs (all of which can present challenges to treatment planning), chart review and history take on special importance. During the chart review look for information on the following:

1. Parkinsonian, ataxic, autonomic, and pyramidal features (see Signs above). This information will help the clinician think about classification and about the number of systems involved and therefore the challenges to treatment planning and success.
2. Note duration of illness, because with increasing duration dysphagia is more likely.
3. Record onset and type of swallowing impairment as reported by others. Ideally, it makes sense to begin managing dysphagia as soon after its appearance as possible to see if some health consequences can be delayed or prevented.
4. Presence of cognitive changes, especially frontal executive signs such as reduced attention and ability to switch tasks, which can influence what rehabilitation can accomplish and may even direct treatment to a degree, should be noted.
5. Behavioral changes related to apathy, depression, and perhaps other variables should be noted, as should the success of any medical treatments aimed at them.
6. The effect and duration of levodopa responsiveness should be recorded.

7. Also note history of previous health consequences, such as aspiration pneumonia, the need for the Heimlich maneuver, and weight loss that may implicate swallowing and add special urgency to management as well as signal future recurrences if management is unsuccessful.

8. Autonomic deficits such as constipation and postural hypotension should be noted. Both interact with diet and posture and may influence what a clinician does. For example, thickened liquids that are often barely tolerated by patients because of taste or feel may be associated with dehydration, which can further complicate constipation.

9. A good history from the patient and caregiver is as critical in this group of conditions as in any other. The history as previously described in Chapter 4 will suffice in MSA. Of special interest are:

   a. Patient's recognition of dysphagia, confirmed or elaborated by family/caregivers.

   b. Influence of dysphagia on quality of life, which can easily be measured by SWAL-QOL (see Appendix A).

   c. Description of any conditions that make swallowing better or worse.

   d. Desire to eat.

   e. Physical ability to eat independently, involving ability to cut food, load a utensil, and move food to the mouth; use a cup, glass and straw; and ability to chew.

   f. Adequacy of saliva. Dry mouth can be frequent.

   g. Influence of dysphagia on health.

   h. Health and ability of family/caregiver(s) to provide assistance.

   i. Signs of apathy or depression.

Clinical Swallow Examination (CSE)

See Chapter 5 for a thorough discussion of the CSE. Pay special attention when examining the MSA patient to the following:

1. Signs in oral nonverbal performance on tests of maximum performance such as alternate motion rates (AMRs), akinesia of speech (impaired movement initiation), weakness, rigidity, spasticity, and incoordination. If incoordination predominates, then improved skill may be most appropriate; if weakness predominates, then some strengthening program may be most sensible. Akinesia will influence treatment decisions as outlined below, and spasticity may make some treatments, such as the Showa, inappropriate because of their potential to further increase abnormal tone.

2. Sign of stridor and its severity.

3. Upper extremity integrity in getting food and drink prepared and into mouth.

4. General cognitive integrity.

5. Evidence of impaired interest, initiation, and intention.

6. Determination of apathy (see Appendix C).

7. Relative integrity of jaw, lips, tongue, palate, larynx, and respiratory mechanism.

Videofluoroscopic Swallow Examination (VFSE)

See Chapter 6 for full details. Of special interest in MSA will be the following:

1. Interpretation of structure movement and bolus flow in support of hypotheses about whether signs

suggest incoordination, lack of initiation, abnormal tone, or weakness is important. Admittedly, these distinctions are difficult but should not be avoided. Treatments without the guidance of at least a hypothesis about the underlying pathophysiology are likely to be misapplied and the negative and even positive effects less informative than they might otherwise be.

2. Pay special attention to hyolaryngeal movement and relationship to UES duration and extent of opening and to the relationship of both to arrival of the bolus. In the absence of manometry, such observations may help the clinician decide if the problem is a failure of UES musculature to relax or if the problem is one of incoordination.

3. Presence and severity of penetration and aspiration.

4. Effect of bolus and posture manipulations.

Videoendoscopic Swallow Examination

See Chapter 7 for more complete details on this exam. Chapter 15 may also be of value when parkinsonian signs and symptoms are prominent. Videoendoscopy may be especially valuable in patients with MSA to confirm laryngeal integrity due to the common stridor in this population. If present, possible determination of whether this movement abnormality appears to be the result of dystonia or weakness may be valuable in management.

Treatment

General treatment principles and principles of compensatory and rehabilitative

techniques plus full descriptions of the techniques themselves appear in Chapters 11–14. This section is limited to a guide to particular compensatory and rehabilitative techniques to consider. Early identification of MSA and early intervention when dysphagia is reported or detected may be especially important. Rapid deterioration is the norm in these conditions, and the health consequences of dysphagia, if not reduced, can hasten decline. A minor but potentially important reason for aggressive rehabilitation is that coughing as can happen with aspiration may cause potentially dangerous hypotension.

Compensatory Approaches

Food and Liquid Preparation. Preserving enjoyment while increasing safety is difficult, although changing food texture is probably less risky than thickening liquids. Any change in liquid viscosity that makes liquids unappealing is likely to lead to noncompliance and/or dehydration. Added moisture is likely to be especially important in those with autonomic failure and subsequent dry mouth. Work with dietetics, pharmacy, and the physician to make sure foods and medications are complementary. If interest and initiation are a problem, then the most flavorable and visually appealing food possible may be important.

Postural Adjustments. *Anterocollis* (the head and neck are held in forward flexion due to increased tone of anterior cervical muscles) is a relatively frequent sign and may actually be therapeutic, as it can resemble the chin down posture. All other postural adjustments are worth evaluating simultaneously with rehabilitation techniques.

Rehabilitation Techniques

Understanding the underlying pathophysiology is especially critical in a condition where that pathophysiology can be so varied. A rigid akinetic state leads to some of the treatment considerations described below. However, ataxia and hypertonicity can also be the main explanations in some patients.

Intention treatment (see p. 106) may be a good first approach if akinesia dominates. Attention treatment (see p. 106) may be a good first approach if attention is disturbed. Combining these two approaches may also be logical. Any of the skill-based treatments such as the Showa or other hard swallow variations (p. 103 and 104) may be useful when incoordination predominates.

If weakness is a major contributor to signs, then one or more of the strengthening treatments may be appropriate, including RMST (p. 83), lingual strengthening (p. 88), and the Shaker head raise exercise (p. 97). If posterior tongue movement is reduced, then the Masako maneuver (p. 101) and other tongue back exercises (p. 111) may be appropriate. Often, combinations of these and other approaches will make for the most efficient treatment package.

SUMMARY

Swallowing problems are frequently encountered and can be expected in patients with MSA. Dysphagia is increasingly viewed as a serious consequence of this condition that may contribute to death. Early identification and management of dysphagia in patients with this condition appears sensible.

17 Other Parkinsonian Syndromes

(Progressive Supranuclear Palsy and Corticobasal Ganglionic Degeneration)

A variety of *atypical parkinsonian syndromes*, different from PD and of which MSA is only one, have been identified. The two to be emphasized in this chapter are *progressive supranuclear palsy* (PSP) and *corticobasal ganglionic degeneration* (CBGD). Oertel & Moller (2004) identify eight other "rare degenerative syndromes associated with parkinsonism":

1. *Frontotemporal dementia and parkinsonism linked to chromosome 17* (FTDP 17), a condition in which parkinsonian features coexist with cognitive and behavioral abnormalities such as excessive eating or *hyperphagia*, conditions that can worsen the results of coexisting dysphagia or suggest dysphagia to the uninitiated.

2. *Pantothenate kinase-associated neurodegeneration* (PKAN), also known by the now-avoided name of *Hallervorden-Spatz syndrome*, a condition that usually appears in childhood characterized by parkinsonian features, including rigidity, pyramidal tract signs such as spasticity, sometimes dystonia and chorea, and cognitive and behavioral decline.

3. *X-linked dystonia-parkinsonism syndrome* (also known as *Lubag* or *Lubag syndrome*), a condition primarily of men from a particular region of the Philippines, characterized most notably by dystonia, which may begin focally and evolve into a generalized dystonia. Parkinsonian features often occur late.

4. *Chorea-acanthocytosis* (CHAC) is frequently characterized by dyskinesias of the face and tongue and chorea of the limbs. Rigidity and other parkinsonian features may occur early or late. Swallowing abnormality is apparently frequent.

5. *Pallidonigroluysian degeneration* (PNLD) is a highly variable disorder in which parkinsonian features may occur along with a number of other abnormal movement patterns. Again, dysphagia requiring management can be posited.

6. *Pallidopyramidal disease* is another of the inherited diseases, usually of young adults, characterized by parkinsonian and pyramidal signs.

7. *Rett's syndrome* is a disorder usually of females with very early onset, characterized by slowed development

often after a short period of reasonably normal development, dementia, and movement abnormalities.

8. *Dementia with Lewy bodies* is a dementing illness in which parkinsonian motor signs can precede intellectual decline or more frequently follow the onset of dementia. Dysphagia can occur and may well contribute to morbidity and mortality.

Not much is known about the dysphagia in these conditions, even less about the appropriate compensations or rehabilitative approaches. However, if referred, the dysphagia clinician should feel compelled to evaluate and treat according to general principles. Despite our ignorance about these conditions, they are mentioned to remind readers of the inadequacy of including only one or a few diagnoses. When dealing with children and adults with parkinsonian conditions, an active practitioner is frequently forced to rely on experience and principles because data are nonexistent.

Before discussing PSP and CBGD, two further introductory comments are necessary for the modern practitioner. First, a shift conceptually away from classifying these conditions as parkinsonian syndromes, with emphasis on the motor deficits, and toward frontotemporal dementia (FTD) syndromes with an emphasis on localization and higher cortical dysfunction, is now underway (Baak, 2008). For readers interested in discussions of these conditions within the rubric of FTD, a book edited by Hodges (2007) makes interesting reading. Because of our emphasis on the motor, specifically swallowing, abnormalities in these conditions, however, we have chosen to stick with the more traditional classifica-

tion. Second, so-called *overlap syndromes* in which characteristics from two or more syndromes may be encountered in the same patient. Nowhere, perhaps, is overlap more common than in those disorders characterized by mixes of parkinsonism and cognitive, linguistic, and behavioral abnormalities. Furthermore, a patient may fit one diagnostic category at one point in his clinical course and evolve into another diagnosis over time. PSP and CBGD, the major focuses of this chapter, are sometimes present as overlaps. As an example of evolution, the form of frontotemporal dementia called *progressive nonfluent aphasia* (PNFA) can evolve into a full-blown CBGD over time. Other examples abound.

What is the clinician to do? We recommend relying upon clinical presentation. An exact diagnosis may be impossible in many cases, though dysphagia assessment and treatment may often be indicated regardless.

PROGRESSIVE SUPRANUCLEAR PALSY

Definition

PSP, also called *Steele-Richardson-Olszewski syndrome*, is a progressive neurologic disorder with its origin usually in middle age. Golbe (2004) has reviewed a substantial portion of the PSP literature and characterizes the condition as usually beginning with difficulty walking accompanied by frequent falls. Patients often develop rigidity, generalized motor and cognitive slowness, dysarthria, dysphagia, visual disturbances, and often but not inevitably vertical gaze palsy. As the disease progresses, patients often have a wide-eyed and astonished expression. Failure to respond to levodopa is also contributory to confident diagnosis. Dystonia is a frequent sign. The differentiation of PSP and PD can be difficult, especially in the early stage of the disease. Differentiation from dementia may also be difficult in that relatively small portion of PSP patients presenting with early behavioral and cognitive changes (Kaat et al., 2007).

Signs/Diagnostic Criteria

A consensus committee has developed diagnostic criteria (Litvan et al., 1996). The diagnosis of possible PSP is based on gradual onset of neurologic symptoms in a person 40 or more years old who has either a vertical gaze palsy alone or in combination with abnormally slow vertical saccades, postural instability, and frequent falls. Supportive criteria are rigidity or akinesia, abnormal neck posture, early onset dysarthria or dysphagia, poor response to dopaminergic medications, and early cognitive changes such as apathy. PSP is the probable diagnosis if age of onset, gaze palsy, postural instability, and frequent falls within the first year of onset are all present. Hyperextension of the neck may also occur and complicate the swallow, reducing the amount and duration of UES opening.

Epidemiology

Onset of PSP is usually between 55 and 70 but has occurred in persons in their 40s. Prevalence is estimated at 3.9 per 100,000 persons in the American popula-

tion (Golbe, 1994). Incidence is reported by Diroma and colleagues (2003) to be 0.3 to 1.1 per 100,000 persons per year. Litvan and colleagues (1996) posit that this prevalence is probably an underestimation because of frequent misdiagnosis. Death after diagnosis can range from 1 to 17 years, with most dying between approximately 5 and 7 years (Litvan et al., 1996). Approximately 30% of PSP patients survive 10 years after diagnosis (Golbe, 2004).

Evaluation

Evaluation begins with a medical history and physical, usually neurologic, examination. The signs mentioned above are what are looked for. In addition to the exam, imaging may serve to rule out other etiologies of change, including stroke and tumor. Imaging is usually not confirmatory of PSP. In this regard, however, it is important to recognize that vascular PSP has been reported (Josephs, Ishizawa, Tsuboi, Cookson, & Dickson, 2002). Neuropsychological examination can establish the presence and severity of behavioral and cognitive changes.

Medical/Surgical Management

Medical and surgical treatments have been generally unsuccessful in PSP. Some signs such as dystonia may be helped with botulinum toxin. The result is that any influence on the functional decline of men and women with PSP will need to be provided by physical, occupational, speech, swallowing, and other therapists.

SWALLOWING IN PSP

Epidemiology

Disordered swallowing, like dysarthria, occurs in PSP and is often a very early sign. Diroma and colleagues (2003) report bulbar signs of dysarthria, dysphonia, and dysphagia as being present at diagnosis in 9 of 25 patients (36%); subsequently, 18 of the 25 (72%) went on to develop dysphagia. Litvan, Sastry, & Sonies (1997) identified dysphagia in 26 of 27 individuals with PSP (96%) based on rigorous testing. Oral stage abnormalities may be more frequent and severe than pharyngeal deficits and may occur earlier. The proportion of PSP patients with dysphagia will vary with duration and severity of disease and with method of test and rigor of interpretation of test performance. Muller and colleagues (2001) report a median duration of disease prior to appearance of dysphagia of 42 months. They describe prognosis after onset of dysphagia as poor and urge early identification and treatment. Dysphagia is probably nearly inevitable at some time in the disease's course, and aspiration pneumonia is a frequent cause of death.

Symptoms

Patients with PSP may be better able to report symptoms than those with PD, even when they present with cognitive impairments (Muller et al., 2001). Thus, providing the patient a chance to report symptoms is critical and SWAL-QOL (Appendix A) includes a list of symptoms, as well as a five-point scoring system for indicating frequency of each. Neumann

and colleagues (1996) report the following most frequent swallowing symptoms:

1. Coughing and choking episodes
2. Difficulty with chewing
3. Drooling
4. Rapid drinking
5. Mouth stuffing

Other symptoms might include:

1. Food building up in the cheeks (Sonies, 1992)
2. Difficulty picking up food from plate
3. Inappropriately large boluses and difficulty moving food into the mouth, both of these because of the gaze palsy that often accompanies this condition

Litvan and colleagues (1997) used a 20-item questionnaire to allow patients to identify their symptoms. All 27 of their patients had at least one symptom, and the average number for the group was 6.6. Interestingly, severity of cognitive impairment (severely cognitively impaired patients were not included) was positively related to number of symptoms reported. The rank order of symptoms reported by their group is displayed in Table 17–1.

Signs

Oral Stage

The following are typical oral stage signs:

1. Poor bolus control
2. "[P]osterior leakage" (Neumann et al., 1996, p. 164)
3. Abnormal posterior tongue movement
4. Delayed initiation of the swallow
5. Ineffective anterior munching

Table 17–1. Swallowing symptoms reported by 27 patients with PSP based on a 20-item questionnaire

Symptom	Percent of Patients Reporting
Coughing or choking while swallowing	74.0
Excessive saliva or mucus in mouth	63.0
Difficulty swallowing	55.6
Food falls out of mouth	55.6
Food gets stuck in cheek	48.1
Slow eater	44.4
Food spreads all over mouth	44.4
Avoids foods like apples, nuts, and cookies	40.7
More difficulty swallowing liquids than solids	37.0
Very dry mouth	33.3
Can't chew hard foods	25.9
Food gets caught at base of tongue	25.9
Can't chew fibrous or "crunchy" foods	25.9
Avoids food like celery	22.2
Food gets caught lower in throat	22.2
Food or water comes into mouth without vomiting, often while lying down	22.2
More difficulty swallowing solids than liquids	18.5
"Lump" in throat	14.8
Food comes out of nose or mouth	11.1
Pain while swallowing	3.7

Note. From "Characterizing Swallowing Abnormalities in Progressive Supra-nuclear Palsy," by I. Litvan, N. Sastry, and B. C. Sonies, 1997, *Neurology, 48,* pp. 1654–1662. Copyright 1997 by Lippincott, Williams & Wilkins. Reprinted with permission.

6. Forceful lingual pressing or "mashing" of food against the hard palate
7. Delayed or uncoordinated lingual movements
8. Noncohesive bolus transfer
9. Absent velar elevation
10. Excessive posterior lingual bolus leakage
11. Delayed swallow onset (Leopold & Kagel, 1997)

Litvan and colleagues (1997), using both VFSE and ultrasound, identify the following:

1. Prolonged oral stage
2. "Impaired tongue motility" (p. 1656)
3. Delayed initiation of the swallow

Pharyngeal Stage

Pharyngeal stage signs include:

1. "Decreased pharyngeal contraction" (Neumann et al., 1996, p. 164)
2. Vallecular retention
3. Pyriform sinus retention
4. Copious, tenacious pharyngeal secretions (Leopold & Kagel, 1997)
5. Greater residual in valleculae than in pyriform sinuses (Litvan et al., 1997), a condition commonly thought to reflect reduced tongue control

Based on EMG assessment, Alfonsi and colleagues (2007) identify a failure of UES relaxation during the pharyngeal stage of swallowing as characteristic of PSP (as well as MSA). This condition could well explain residual in the pyriform sinuses and aspiration after the swallow.

Laryngeal Stage

Typical laryngeal stage signs are the following:

1. Penetration was identified by Leopold and Kagel (1997) as supraglottic and glottic.
2. Aspiration was identified in some patients by Neumann and colleagues (1996), but Leopold and Kagel (1997) say they observed no frank penetration.

3. Litvan and colleagues (1997) identified aspiration in only 5 of their 27 patients (19%). Nonetheless, the clinician should have a high degree of suspicion about the possibility of aspiration in this population.

Functional/Quality of Life Consequences

None has been established experimentally, but any of the generally expected consequences on function and health can be expected. More specifically to PSP, when paralysis of downward gaze is part of the syndrome, eating can be especially challenging and may be unpleasant. Not being able to see what is on the plate easily, nor to see what is being loaded on a utensil or cut up, can destroy pleasure and threaten adequacy and safety. Awareness of these difficulties is generally preserved in PSP, so that patients do not have even the protection that comes with lack of insight.

Health Consequences

Aspiration pneumonia is a frequent cause of death. Malnutrition and even dehydration can occur. Golbe (2004) recommends percutaneous endoscopic gastrostomy (PEG) after the first aspiration pneumonia, when eating takes longer than the family can accommodate, when substantial weight loss occurs because of malnutrition, and when some aspiration occurs with every bolus.

Swallowing Evaluation

Because of the risk of morbidity and mortality from dysphagia in this population, early referral and careful examination and treatment can be critical.

Chart Review and History

Chapter 4 contains a thorough discussion of these components of the evaluation. These patients are often capable of giving a reasonably complete history. Of special interest will be:

1. Any data that increase the probability of the appropriateness of the diagnosis (see Signs above)
2. Duration of disease
3. Presence, time of onset, course, and present severity of dysphagia
4. Any special difficulty with eating or drinking
5. Health consequences of dysphagia
6. Evidence of behavioral or cognitive involvement
7. Any report of functional consequences of eating
8. Any report of special adaptations patient or family has made to how or what is taken for nutrition and hydration
9. Caregiver role in keeping patient adequately nourished and safe
10. Advanced directives about nonoral nutrition and hydration

Clinical Swallow Examination (CSE

The CSE is thoroughly discussed in Chapter 5. Of special importance is an observation of independent eating and drinking to determine adequacy and safety. Experimentation with special utensils, food positioning, or method of supplying liquids (e.g., special cups) is also important to determine effect on adequacy and safety of eating.

Videofluoroscopic Swallow Examination (VFSE)

Procedures for the VFSE are completely described in Chapter 6. Of special interest in PSP are the following:

1. Careful comparison of oral and pharyngeal stages, as the former is more likely to be involved than the latter at least early in the disease.
2. Contrast of clinician and patient supplied boluses, with every attempt to approximate the selection and delivery of solids and liquids done at home. We recognize this can only be a gross approximation, even under the best of conditions.
3. Data in support of the strongest possible hypothesis about whether signs are related to weakness, rigidity, dystonia, or some other muscle or movement abnormality. This may be especially important for the UES, where failure to relax is a frequent but not inevitable finding.
4. Analysis of poor bolus control and of the "mashing" that Leopold and Kagel (1997) described.
5. Data in support of the strongest possible hypothesis about the safest bolus types and sizes for both solids and liquids.
6. Data in support of therapeutic effects of postural adjustments, especially on penetration and aspiration.

Videoendoscopic Swallow Examination

Complete details on the use of videoendoscopy in dysphagia assessment with movement disorders patients are found in Chapter 7. Chapter 15 may provide some additional guidance when features of parkinsonism are thought to be influencing the swallow.

TREATMENT

Compensatory Approaches

In the absence of any data on effect on swallowing of rehabilitation or perhaps because of persisting nihilism about rehabilitation, most general discussions review compensations and tube placement. Any of the compensations described in Chapter 13 could be employed, and we will describe one or two specific ones below. However, we again want to make it clear that these methods are most appropriate only if rehabilitation has failed or if they occur simultaneously with rehabilitation. Specific approaches may be prompted by at least a portion of those with PSP, such as:

1. Experimentation with food placement to accommodate the gaze paralysis when it is present. This may mean placing food and drink on a surface whose height can be increased to make looking down less necessary.
2. Smaller portions and even multiple small meals may also help control maladaptive eating behaviors.
3. Urge adequate hydration to help control the copious secretions identified by Leopold and Kagel (1997).
4. Referral for the best possible fitting of dentures or partials in the case of missing teeth, especially posterior in the mouth, is always a good idea and may be especially important in those with PSP, whom Leopold and Kagel (1997) described as having ineffective anterior chewing patterns.
5. Recall that Litvan and colleagues (1997) report the frequent complaint by patients of difficulty chewing. Softer food, more moisture, and dropping difficult foods whose tex-

ture cannot be modified may also be important.

Rehabilitation Techniques

Chapter 14 contains complete descriptions of the major treatment approaches used for dysphagia, regardless of etiology. Some of those that may be of particular interest for persons with PSP are described below. Interestingly, however, no specific methodology for the chewing abnormality described by Leopold and Kagel (1997) has been reported, despite the probable frequency of this abnormality in neurologic disease. It may well be that this problem is not treatable, but we would certainly try to direct those patients to chew with more vigor and reinforce them if they did so. Otherwise, the clinician will have to resort to attempted rehabilitation of the rest of the swallowing mechanism. Although the whole array of treatments described in Chapter 14 may be appropriate, those that focus on the oral stage may be most successful.

Intention treatment (see p. 106) may be a good first treatment for those patients with prolonged inactivity during the oral stage or who have inefficient swallowing. Sensory stimulation in the form of thermal tactile application (TTA; see p. 110) may also be tried, especially for those with long delays in oral initiation of the swallow. LSVT (see p. 81) has been of demonstrated effect in PD and may be appropriate here. Variations of the hard swallow (see p. 104) may have a positive influence on oral stage function. The Masako maneuver (see p. 101), hawk technique, or other posterior tongue maneuvers (see p. 111) may also be of worth.

If airway closure is a problem, then the supraglottic swallow (see p. 99) may be appropriate. If UES opening is reduced, then the Shaker head raise exercise (see p. 97) and the Mendelsohn maneuver (see p. 94) may be indicated

Summary

Dysphagia occurs commonly in individuals with PSP. Data on treatment effects in PSP are nonexistent; however, the clinician should not be dissuaded. Logical techniques are available. If patients, family/caregivers, and medical teams are willing to take a chance, then treatment may reward that willingness.

CORTICOBASAL GANGLIONIC DEGENERATION

Definition

CBGD, also called corticobasal degeneration, corticobasal syndrome, or corticobasal degeneration syndrome, is a sporadic, neurodegenerative disease of unknown etiology beginning typically with unilateral rigidity and bradykinesia that are unresponsive to dopaminergic medications. Tremor is mild or absent in most cases. As Bak (2008) observes, the hallmark of the condition is its heterogeneity. However, in addition to the signs of parkinsonism, cortical abnormalities are likely and can include dementia, alien limb phenomenon, cortical sensory loss, and, as the bulbar musculature becomes involved, apraxia of speech and dysphagia. The *alien limb phenomenon* is dramatic when it occurs and involves some element of movement independent of the patient's will and sometimes even awareness. Fernandez and colleagues

(2007) describe alien limb as having a feeling of foreignness about the movements of the limb. A variety of other signs may appear, including limb apraxia, oral and speech apraxia, myoclonus, dystonia, and choreoathetosis. CBGD is one of the tauopathies, which is to say that signs result from abnormal accumulations of the protein tau. Other tauopathies include Pick's disease, varieties of FTD, and PSP. Separation of these conditions clinically can be difficult. Differential diagnosis of CBGD and other disorders combining movement and cognitive abnormalities such as Alzheimer's disease, Parkinson's disease with dementia, and dementia with Lewy bodies can be especially difficult.

Signs and Diagnostic Criteria

The condition typically begins unilaterally with clumsiness, rigidity, and/or akinesia. The signs are generally unresponsive to levodopa, and extension to bilateral involvement usually occurs within months to 1 year. Cortical signs can occur early or late and include limb, oral, and speech apraxia; aphasia; cortical sensory abnormalities such as astereognosis; and frontal release signs such as abnormal oral reflexes or a *Myerson's sign* (inability to inhibit the blink when having one's forehead rhythmically tapped). A variety of neuropsychiatric signs can also occur including depression, irritability, apathy, and even disinhibition and obsessive-compulsive disorder. Litvan and colleagues (2003) have identified the following as signaling a probable diagnosis of CBGD: asymmetric onset and one or more cortical signs such as alien limb or apraxia of limbs or bulbar musculature, akinetic-rigid parkinsonism, and lack of response to levodopa, accompanied by dystonia and/

or myoclonus. Neuropathologic criteria for a diagnosis of CBGD have been proposed by Dickson and colleagues (2002).

Brain imaging is often normal in the condition's early stages, but with progression, unilateral atrophy greatest in frontal and parietal cortices is often identified. The most involved hemisphere is likely that contralateral to the side of onset of motor signs. When aphasia is present, the involvement is likely to extend into the temporal lobe on the left. Atrophy may be more likely in the frontal lobe if apraxia is a major sign and in the parietal and temporal lobes if aphasia is predominant.

Evolution

According to Stover, Wainer, & Watts (2004), CBGD becomes bilateral and debilitating in 5 to 10 years. Declines in motor, cognitive, and neuropsychiatric signs do not necessarily parallel one another, and disabling cognitive or motor signs may predominate. In our experience, mutism often occurs late, as does life-threatening dysphagia. According to Stover et al. (2004), bilateral motor signs and signs of frontal lobe abnormality are associated with a more precipitous disease course. Dysphagia related complications often contribute to death. Wenning and colleagues (1998) report a range of survival after onset of disease of 2.5 to 12.5 years, with bilateral slowness and frontal lobe signs having the poorest prognosis.

Epidemiology

The condition is rare, although Stover and colleagues (2004) suspect the diagnosis is often not appreciated. Onset is usually after age 60, but cases in their fourth decade have been confirmed. The condition may be more frequent in women and seems to be idiopathic without a history of inheritance.

Evaluation

A thorough clinical evaluation of movement, cognitive, and psychiatric variables can establish the possible or probable presence of the disorder. Imaging can also contribute to diagnosis. The condition can be confirmed at autopsy with evidence of abnormal aggregations of tau. The criteria for diagnosing these three conditions are adapted from Litvan and colleagues (2003) and are provided here to help clinicians begin to think about differentiating the varieties of patients they may be seeing.

Treatment

Medical and surgical treatments appear to have limited or no influence on signs in CBGD. Dopaminergic medications may influence the parkinsonian signs in a limited number of cases (Kompoliti et al., 1998). Fernandez and colleagues (2007) recommend medications for depression, myoclonus, and spasm.

SWALLOWING IN CBGD

Epidemiology

Dysphagia occurs frequently in CBGD. Muller and colleagues (2001) say that "subjective" dysphagia, by which they mean it was included in the examining neurologist's medical note as having been reported by the patient, occurs within a year of the appearance of dysarthria, an observation perhaps influenced by the fact that dysarthria is easier to identify clinically than dysphagia. Those authors report that it occurred in 31% of their 13 patients on average 64 months following diagnosis. This is, on average, earlier than in PD but does not distinguish CBGD from MSA, PSP, and DLB. The appearance of dysphagia suggests a shortened life expectancy, and death from dysphagia-related medical conditions is frequent. Mahapatra and colleagues (2004) call dysphagia "an important late-presenting symptom" (p. 741) whose presence and management are critical to prolonged life. Unfortunately, reports of careful examination of the swallowing mechanism are rare, and so we are forced to rely on clinical experience and intuition.

Symptoms

These probably vary according to the mix of behavioral, movement, cognitive, and other higher cortical dysfunction in the individual patients. Frattali and Sonies (2000) used a swallowing questionnaire to guide interviews with 15 CBGD patients and their caregivers. Much of what follows is taken from their report (see Table 17–2).

Another way to think about symptoms is in relationship to the predominant cognitive, motor, and behavioral features of the individual patient. If frontal disinhibition predominates, then rapid eating of inappropriately large boluses, excessive eating, or other eating abnormalities may occur. If rigidity and bradykinesia predominate, then slow, inadequate chew-

ing and bolus formation and movement may occur, as may other signs as outlined in Chapter 15 on PD. Choking and coughing may occur in any presentation of the disorder. In other words, heterogeneity is likely to be the norm.

Many CBGD patients seem to be remarkably aware of their difficulties (Bak, 2008), which may lead to extreme care during eating and drinking. However, it is important to note that Frattali and Sonies (2000) report that caregiver report was more consistent with objective signs derived from VFSE than were the patients', who tended to underreport symptoms.

Signs

Frattali and Sonies (2000) have published one of the few systematic evaluations of swallowing in CBGD. The signs to be listed are drawn from their work.

Oral Stage

Oral stage signs included:

1. Piecemeal deglutition, in which bolus is divided into small portions prior to swallow initiation
2. Delay in initiation of the swallow
3. "Excessive lingual gestures" (p. 157)
4. Impaired posterior movement of the bolus
5. Nasal regurgitation

Pharyngeal Stage

Pharyngeal stage signs included:

1. Pooling in the valleculae
2. Pooling in pyriform sinuses
3. Entry of the bolus deep into the pharynx prior to swallow initiation

Table 17–2. Swallowing symptoms, as reported by patients and families and their frequency for 14 persons with CBGD

Symptom	Number of Participants out of 14
Difficulty swallowing	12 (86%)
Coughing/choking	11 (79%)
Slow eater	9 (64%)
More difficulty with liquids than solids	7 (50%)
Difficulty swallowing pills	7 (50%)
Food spreading over mouth	6 (43%)
Food stuck in cheek and not swallowed	6 (43%)
Dry mouth	6 (43%)
Food falling from mouth	5 (36%)
Food caught lower in throat	4 (29%)
Feeling of lump in throat	3 (21%)
Difficulty chewing foods	3 (21%)
Avoiding foods	3 (21%)
Food coming out of nose	3 (21%)
Food caught at base of tongue	3 (21%)
Reflux	2 (14%)
More difficulty with solids than liquids	2 (14%)

Note. From "Speech and Swallowing Disturbances in Corticobasal Degeneration," by C. M. Frattali and B. C. Sonies, 2000, in: I. Litvan, C. G. Goetz, and A. E. Lang (Eds.), *Advances in Neurology, 82,* pp. 153–160. Copyright 2000 by Lippincott, Williams & Wilkins. Reprinted with permission.

Laryngeal Stage

Laryngeal stage signs included:

1. Both penetration and aspiration.
2. Penetration occurred more frequently than aspiration.

Functional/Quality of Life Consequences

No study documenting these influences is known to us. However, one can predict the potential of the full range of such consequences. Given that rehabilitation of the swallow is seldom mentioned, Stover et al. (2004) being a notable exception, and that the majority of writers appear to feel that diet change, other compensations, and tube feeding are the only alternatives if patients are to remain safe and well nourished, one can predict that patients so treated experience and suffer, as a minimum:

1. Loss of autonomy
2. Loss of the enjoyment of eating and drinking
3. Feelings of being inadequately nourished and hydrated despite laboratory values to the contrary
4. Loss of socialization around mealtime and other family and friend events
5. Changes in role within the family, as carving the turkey at holiday time loses its allure if one is eating puree or taking nutrition via tube

Health Consequences

The dangers of aspiration are highlighted by nearly all writers, and death hastened by the consequences of aspiration is frequent. One can speculate that malnutrition and dehydration are also frequent unless a patient has a capable and concerned caregiver.

Swallowing Evaluation

History and Chart Review

Chapter 4 describes generic histories and chart reviews. Of special interest in CBGD are:

1. Duration of condition.

2. Presenting signs. This is especially important as those signs will provide hints about differential diagnosis, which can be so complex in this condition.
3. More particularly, any information on the type and severity of motor, cognitive, and behavioral abnormalities. Intact cognition and behavior make for a brighter prognosis for rehabilitation efforts. Impaired cognition or behavior may explain critical signs, such as overeating or hyperphagia (rapid eating) and other behaviors that threaten health even in the presence of an adequate swallow.
4. Any observations of eating and drinking behaviors.
5. Differential diagnosis. Differential diagnosis can be very difficult, and often the best that one can hope for is a short list of diagnostic possibilities with associated probabilities.
6. Any indication of physician's knowledge about dysphagia and attitudes about rehabilitation, compensations, and tube feeding.

Clinical Swallow Examination (CSE)

The traditional examination is fully described in Chapter 5. Of particular interest in CBGD are:

1. Observation of one or more meals to look for behavioral abnormalities that may complicate the motor act of swallowing
2. Observation of limb apraxia or alien limb, which may disrupt ability for patients to feed themselves
3. Evidence of insight into eating or swallowing abnormalities; insight is a predictor of response to rehabilita-

tion and even to suggested compensations

4. Documentation of any compensations that seem to be associated with safer, more efficient eating and drinking without posing too serious a threat to quality of life

5. Documentation of cognitive, behavioral, and motor abnormalities present during or likely to influence safe, adequate, and pleasurable nutrition and hydration

Videofluoroscopic Swallow Examination (VFSE)

The complete examination is described in Chapter 6. If a patient's symptoms are primarily parkinsonian, Chapter 15 may also provide some guidance. Other considerations include:

1. Ability to provide and swallow boluses without assistance from the clinician may be informative.

2. Similarly, cognitive and behavioral abnormalities should prompt an atypical portion of the exam in which the opportunity to display the threat to safety of typical eating behaviors is provided. This can be unnerving to the traditional clinician and may be prohibited in some centers. If so, the CSE or a complete history will need to be substituted.

3. The effect of compensatory and rehabilitative techniques should, as always, be estimated during the VFSE.

Videoendoscopic Swallow Examination

Complete details on the use of the videoendoscopic exam can be found in Chapter 7 and Chapter 15 may be of additional value when parkinsonian signs and symptoms predominate.

Treatment

Compensations

The full range of compensations outlined in Chapter 13 may apply, and that chapter should be consulted. However, the frequent occurrence of frontal lobe cognitive and neuropsychiatric abnormalities in this population may prompt more heroic measures. For example:

1. Portions may have to be severely restricted to prevent gorging.
2. Full-time supervision may be necessary.
3. Traditional compensations such as changing food texture and liquid viscosity or altering posture may simply not be possible.

Rehabilitation

To the degree that motor symptoms predominate, the full range of rehabilitation techniques from Chapter 14 may be tried, consistent with the presumed underlying pathophysiology and the type and distribution of the oral and pharyngeal stage abnormalities and penetration and aspiration events. Because the motor deficits are likely to be rigidity, bradykinesia, weakness, difficulty with initiation, and perhaps even apraxia, the following may be useful:

1. Respiratory muscle strength training (RMST) (p. 83)
2. Lingual strength training (p. 88)
3. LSVT (p. 81)
4. Hard (effortful) swallow in all its permutations (p. 104)
5. Intention/attention treatment (p. 106)

6. Mendelsohn maneuver (p. 94)
7. Supraglottic swallow (p. 99)
8. Masako maneuver (p. 101)
9. Showa maneuver (p. 103)

Additionally, dietary consultation is likely to be critical.

Summary

Though dysphagia is to be expected in patients with CBDG, no treatment effect data exist. The heterogeneity of these patients makes it unlikely that clinical trials for dysphagia rehabilitation will ever be completed. Clinicians will have to plan their treatment based on experience and on the best possible characterization of each patient's cluster of motor, cognitive, and neuropsychiatric abnormalities. Prognosis of benefit from treatment is not as good as in PD, but that should not dissuade the practitioner from aggressive rehabilitation attempts.

18 Dystonia

DEFINITION

Dystonia is a heterogeneous condition that results in involuntary, sustained, and often repetitive contractions of opposing muscles resulting in twisting movements and abnormal postures. It is typical to classify dystonia by etiology (i.e., primary or secondary) or distribution (i.e., generalized, segmental, and focal). *Primary dystonia* may occur hereditarily or arise sporadically, while *secondary dystonia* is most commonly associated with other neurologic conditions (e.g., traumatic brain injury, anoxic brain injury). *Generalized dystonia* affects muscles throughout the body. In contrast, *focal dystonia* affects only one body part, such as the neck in cervical dystonia (or spasmodic torticollis) or the eyes in blepharospasm. *Segmental dystonia* affects two or more contiguous body parts, such as the eyes in combination with the lower face, mouth, and/or tongue in oromandibular dystonia (or Meige syndrome). Dystonia may also be classified based on age upon onset (early onset or late onset). Other classification systems and terminology may also be encountered in this complex condition, such as dystonia-plus syndromes (e.g., dopa-responsive dystonia, myoclonus-dystonia syndrome), pseudo-dystonia, and psychogenic dystonia (Fahn, Bressman, & Marsden, 1998; Fernandez, Rodriguez, Skidmore, & Okun, 2007).

SIGNS/DIAGNOSTIC CRITERIA

The main signs are:

1. Twisting movements or abnormal postures of relatively long duration (in comparison to the brief movements encountered in chorea, for example).
2. Simultaneous contraction of opposing muscles in agonist and antagonist muscles in a given body part.
3. Though the involved muscle distribution may vary (and progress) over time, the affected musculature is fairly constant in comparison to the movement abnormalities encountered in patients with chorea.
4. Primary dystonia almost invariably begins with a single body part, often a leg or arm, and then gradually becomes more generalized.
5. Onset in the lower extremities tends to occur in younger individuals and be associated with a greater likelihood of progressing to generalized dystonia.

6. Onset in the upper extremities tends to occur in older individuals and is less likely to progress to generalized dystonia (Greene, Kang, & Fahn, 1995).
7. Age of onset is important prognostically, as dystonia is more likely to become generalized in younger individuals.
8. The use of sensory tricks (*geste antagoniste*) by the patient, such as lightly touching the affected body part, may often provide relief.
9. Signs are typically exacerbated by stress or fatigue and are relieved by sleep or relaxation.

A variety of rating scales have been developed to aid in the evaluation of dystonia. The *Burke-Fahn-Marsden Scale* is one widely used dystonia scale that evaluates dystonia in nine body areas, including speech and swallowing, using a 0–4 scale with a lower score indicating milder severity (Burke et al., 1985). However, limitations of this scale have been cited, such as the small number of patients included in the initial work and lack of follow-up in multicenter studies.

In response to these limitations, the *Unified Dystonia Rating Scale* (UDRS) was developed. The UDRS rates 14 body areas using a severity and duration rating. Similar to the Burke-Fahn-Marsden Scale, severity is determined for each body region using a 0 (no dystonia) to 4 (extreme dystonia) scale. Duration is rated with a 0–4 scale (with increments of 0.5) based on factors such as the intensity of dystonia and whether it occurs at rest or with action. Table 18–1 summarizes the 14 body areas assessed with the UDRS. The total score reflects a summary of severity and duration scores for all body areas (Comella et al., 2003).

The *Global Dystonia Rating Scale* (GDS) also rates dystonia in the 14 areas of

Table 18–1. Body areas assessed by the Unified Dystonia Rating Scale (UDRS)

Eyes and upper face
Lower face
Jaw and tongue
Larynx
Neck
Shoulder and proximal arm (R and L)
Distal arm and hand including elbow (R and L)
Pelvis and proximal leg (R and L)
Distal leg and foot including knee (R and L)
Trunk

Note. From "Rating Scales for Dystonia: A Multicenter Assessment," by C. L. Comella, S. Leurgans, J. Wuu, G. T. Stebbins, T. Chmure, and the Dystonia Study Group, 2003, *Movement Disorders, 18,* 303–312. Reprinted with permission.

the UDRS, in this case on a 0–10 rating scale. Again, a lower number indicates less severe dystonia in that body area (e.g., 0 = no dystonia in a particular body part, 10 = most severe dystonia in a particular body part) (Comella et al., 2003). Scales aimed at segmental and focal dystonias have been developed as well, such as the *Toronto Western Spasmodic Torticollis Rating Scale* (TWSTRS) for cervical dystonia (Consky, Basinki, Belle, Ranawaya, & Lang, 1990).

EVOLUTION OVER TIME

Signs generally start with a single body part and may progress to a more generalized distribution over time. Age at onset is the most important prognostic factor in the development of additional signs. That is, the younger an individual is at the time of onset, the more likely she is to develop generalized dystonia. Conversely, the older a person is at the time of onset, the more likely that the distribution of affected musculature remains focal or segmental. It has been suggested that 21 years of age is a useful marker to distinguish between early- and late-onset dystonia (Elia et al., 2006; Fahn, Marsden, & Calne, 1987), though others have suggested later markers to distinguish these groups (32 years) (Elia et al., 2006). Onset in the lower extremities is associated with more severe, generalized dystonia in younger patients, while onset in the upper extremities is more likely to occur in older patients and not progress to the generalized form (Greene et al., 1995).

EPIDEMIOLOGY

Primary dystonia is "relatively uncommon," though "the reported prevalence is thought to be underestimated due the lack of identification of patients who have milder symptoms" (Asgeirsson, Jakobsson, Hjaltason, Jonsdottir, & Sveinbjornsdottir, 2006, p. 293), as well as other factors such as the lack of diagnostic markers, the heterogeneity of the condition, and the use of multiple classification systems. Dystonia is being recognized with increasingly regularity over the last decade (Defazio, 2007).

Defazio (2007) summarized 14 published primary dystonia prevalence studies and reported substantial variability, likely due to methodological differences or differences in the characteristics of the study population (e.g., ethnicity, environment, size of population studied). In early-onset dystonia, these prevalence rates ranged from 3 to 50 cases per 1,000,000 and from 30 to 7320 cases per 1,000,000 in late-onset dystonia. Prevalence rates in early-onset dystonia are likely related to ethnicity. For example, Zilber and colleagues (1984) reported a prevalence rate of 24 per 1,000,000 in Israel, Butler et al. (2004) described a prevalence of 40 per 1,000,000 in Northern England, and a prevalence rate of 50 per 1,000,000 has been reported in the Ashkenazi Jews of New York (Risch et al., 1995). Similar variability is found in the prevalence data in patients with late-onset-dystonia: 101 per 1,000,000 in Japan (Matsumoto, Nishimura, Shibasaki, & Kaji, 2003), 136 per 1,000,000 in Serbia (Pekmezovic et al., 2003), 254 per 1,000,000 in Norway (Dung Le, Niulsen, & Dietrichs, 2003), and 430 per 1,000,000 in Northern England (Butler, Duffey, Hawthorne, & Barnes, 2004).

Asgeirsson and colleagues (2003) completed an interesting total population study of primary dystonia in Iceland and found the prevalence for all primary dystonia types to be 37.1 per 1,000,000. As noted by the authors, Iceland offers several interesting scientific considerations for such a study, such as a small population of individuals who share a common ethnic background (99% Caucasian) and a comprehensive system of socialized medicine in which there is only one university-based neurological department. Focal dystonia had a much higher prevalence than segmental or generalized dystonia. Table 18–2 shows the prevalence rates for the focal dystonias reported by these researchers.

The prevalence of focal dystonia is greater than generalized dystonia. Cervical dystonia is the most common form of focal dystonia (Dauer, Burke, Greene, & Fahn, 1998) and commonly appears between the fourth and sixth decades of

Table 18–2. Focal dystonia prevalence rates for focal dystonias in Iceland in 2003

Cervical Dystonia (11.5/1,000,000)

Limb Dystonia (8.0/1,000,000)

Laryngeal Dystonia (5.9/1,000,000)

Blepharospasm (3.1/1,000,000

Oromandibular Dystonia (2.8/1,000,000)

Note. From "Prevalence Study of Primary Dystonia in Iceland," by H. Asgeirsson, F. Jakobsson, H. Hjaltason, H. Jonsdottir, and S. Sveinbjornsdottir, 2006, *Movement Disorders, 21,* pp. 293–298. Reprinted by permission.

life (Duane, 1988). Dystonia occurs more often in women than men (Asgeirsson et al., 2006; Nutt, Muenter, Aronson, Kurland, & Melton, 1988).

MEDICAL/SURGICAL MANAGEMENT

No cure for dystonia is available and treatment generally focuses on symptomatic management. Treatment can be challenging, and multiple approaches are often used in various combinations. Response to treatment varies greatly and results may be unsatisfactory in some cases. Secondary dystonia is generally less responsive to treatment than primary dystonia.

Medical Management

A variety of pharmacological agents have been used in the treatment of dystonia. In most cases, treatment is symptomatic and targets relief of dystonic spasms and pain, though specific therapeutic options

are available for patients with dopa-responsive dystonia and Wilson's disease. Approaches to medical treatment can generally be divided into oral and injectable medications. Oral medications are often the foundation for treatment in patients with early-onset generalized or segmental dystonia, while adult-onset focal dystonia is more commonly treated with botulinum toxin (Bhidayasiri & Tarsy, 2007). This section will be limited to a general listing of the types of these medications. For further details, see Bhidayasiri and Tarsy (2007) and Balash and Giladi (2004).

Oral Medications

Common oral medications used in treatment of dystonia include:

1. Dopaminergic medications (e.g., levodopa, carbidopa)
2. Anticholinergics (e.g., trihexyphenidyl, benzotropine)
3. GABA agonists (e.g., oral baclofen)
4. Antidopaminergic medications (e.g., clozapine, risperidone)
5. Benzodiazepines (e.g., clonazepam, diazepam)

Injectable Medications

These include:

1. GABA agonists (e.g., intrathecal baclofen)
2. Botulinum toxin type A (e.g., Botox, Dysport) and B (e.g., Myobloc)

Surgical Management

The choices are selective peripheral denervation, ablative neurosurgical procedures (including pallidotomy and thalamotomy), and deep brain stimulation (DBS). DBS can be of the internal portion of globus pallidus (GPi) or the ventrolateral thalamus.

Complications

Possibly the most common unwanted result of treatment is poor response to available therapeutics. Oral medications are often prescribed in high dosages and may result in intolerable side effects. Local adverse reactions may occur following treatment with botulinum toxin, usually due to local weakness (Jankovic, 2004). Resistance to botulinum toxin therapy may occur due to the development of antibodies. However, when dosage recommendations are followed and treatment is provided no more frequently than every 3 months, this risk is reduced (Stacy, 2007).

Infection is the most common adverse event associated with DBS in dystonia. Other unwanted reported outcomes include dysarthria, hardware-related problems (e.g., lead fracture or migration), edema, hematoma, and anarthria (Cersosimo et al., 2008; Kupsch et al., 2006; Vidailhet et al., 2005).

The effects of DBS on swallowing function are largely unexplored. Dysphagia has been reported to occur due to stimulation-related muscle contractions in patients with dystonia treated with DBS (Tagliati, Shils, & Alterman, 2004).

Influence on Swallowing

Medical/surgical management of dystonia may result in improved, unchanged, or worsened swallowing function. For example, treatment of cervical dystonia with botulinum toxin may improve posture for safe swallowing but may also result in the onset of dysphagia or an increase in its severity due to weakness. Weakness due to cervical injections may be due to poor selection of targets, injection of unaffected muscles, and diffusion. In severe cases, the requirement of feeding tubes has been reported. Botulinum toxin type B is more commonly associated with dysphagia, possibly due to both weakness and decreased saliva production (Comella et al., 2005; Stacy, 2007).

SWALLOWING IN DYSTONIA

Epidemiology

Due to the heterogeneous nature of the etiology, distribution, and severity of dystonia, it is difficult to determine the prevalence of dysphagia in this population. However, in individuals with spasmodic torticollis, for example, VFSE has revealed oropharyngeal dysphagia in 50% or more of cases (Horner, Riski, Ovelmen-Levitt, & Nashold, 1992; Horner, Riski, Weber, & Nashold, 1993; Riski, Horner, & Nashold, 1990). It appears likely that the prevalence of dysphagia in patients with dystonia increases when the distribution affects musculature involved in swallowing, including the respiratory mechanism.

Symptoms

Much of our knowledge about dysphagia in dystonia comes from studies involving patients with cervical dystonia and oromandibular dystonia. Therefore, the discussion below of the swallowing symptoms and signs will focus on data primarily derived from these populations. However, this is not to suggest that dystonia affecting other portions of the swallowing mechanism will not result in dysphagia. Rather, when the locus of dystonia targets any of the components of the swallowing mechanism, dysphagia may result. Dysphagia may be encountered in generalized dystonia (often due to involvement of the respiratory mechanism), lingual dystonia (including tongue protrusion dystonia) (Schneider et al., 2006), jaw dystonia, and other dystonic conditions.

Cervical Dystonia/Spasmodic Torticollis

Up to two thirds of patients with cervical dystonia may report a subjective complaint of difficulty swallowing, often attributed to abnormal posture. Many individuals who do not report swallowing difficulty will exhibit some degree of dysphagia during instrumental assessment (Horner et al., 1993; Riski et al., 1990). Discomfort with swallowing may be reported (Riski et al., 1990).

Oromandibular Dystonia/Meige Syndrome

Weight loss may be reported, especially in those with orobuccolingual dyskinesias. Treatment with tetrabenazine in conjunction with other medications and/or botulinum toxin may result in weight gain in some cases.

Pain during eating may be experienced. Social embarrassment may also be described (Papapetropoulos & Singer, 2006). A sticking sensation in the throat may be reported. Difficulties with mouth opening and/or tongue movements may be described (Golper, Nutt, Rau, & Coleman, 1983). The subjective report of dys-

phagia may underestimate the presence of difficulty swallowing during instrumental assessment (Cersosimo, Juri, Suárez de Chandler, Clerici, & Micheli, 2005).

Signs

The following list of signs is derived primarily from VFSE, as this procedure has been most frequently used in studies of swallowing in those with dystonia. Signs are divided into oral, pharyngeal, and laryngeal signs, though the reader is again cautioned that these divisions are largely arbitrary.

Cervical Dystonia/Spasmodic Torticollis

Oral Stage. Abnormal bolus preparation may be present (Horner et al., 1992; Riski et al., 1990).

Pharyngeal Stage. Pharyngeal swallow delay is commonly encountered. Postswallow pharyngeal residue, particularly in the valleculae, is also common (Horner et al., 1992; Horner et al., 1993; Riski et al., 1990). Upper esophageal sphincter (UES) dysfunction may be encountered as suggested by the presence of pyriform sinus residue (Riski et al., 1990). Asymmetric bolus transport may be exhibited (Horner et al., 1992; Horner et al., 1993; Riski et al., 1990). Pharyngeal outpouching (*pharyngocele*) may occasionally be encountered (Riski et al., 1990), and this is more common following rhizotomy (Horner et al., 1992).

Laryngeal Stage. Aspiration generally occurs infrequently but it may be encountered (Horner et al., 1992; Riski et al., 1990). Silent aspiration may occur or the cough response may be delayed (Riski et al., 1990). Aspiration is more common following rhizotomy (Horner et al., 1992).

Oromandibular Dystonia/Meige Syndrome

Oral Stage. Premature spillage may be a common finding on VFSE. Cersosimo and colleagues (2005) describe alterations in bolus preparation in surprisingly few patients. Nasal regurgitation may also be encountered less commonly (Cersosimo et al., 2005).

Pharyngeal Stage. Postswallow pharyngeal residue in the valleculae and pyriform sinuses is commonly encountered. Pharyngeal swallow delay may also be encountered. *Pharyngeal lacuna* (a depression at the pharyngeal end of the eustachian tube) is observed rarely. *Aerophagia* (swallowing of air) is also rarely observed (Cersosimo et al., 2005).

Laryngeal Stage. Penetration and aspiration are not commonly reported in the literature (Cersosimo et al., 2005). Our clinical experience suggests that these signs occur less frequently than might be expected.

Functional/QOL Influences

The impact of dysphagia on QOL in patients with dystonia has received little attention in the literature, though Papapetropoulos and Singer (2006) report social embarrassment with eating in patients with oromandibular dystonia. In our clinical experience, patients with dystonia and dysphagia may report other related QOL influences, including:

1. Slowness of eating

2. Decreased enjoyment of eating and drinking
3. "Messy eating" for a variety of reasons
4. Reluctance to eat in public also for a variety of reasons

Health Consequences

The primary health consequence of dysphagia in patients with dystonia appears to be weight loss. Dehydration and malnutrition may also occur.

Swallowing Evaluation

Procedures for the chart review and history, clinical swallow examination (CSE), the videofluoroscopic swallow examination (VFSE), and the videoendoscopic swallow examination appear in Chapters 4, 5, 6, and 7. The emphasis here is on special observations and procedural modifications that might be critical to the best evaluation of swallowing in people with dystonia.

Chart Review and History

As always, a thorough chart review and history is invaluable. Its results will help focus subsequent examinations and provide potentially crucial information to treatment planning. Please see Chapter 4 for more complete details regarding the swallowing history. Items deserving particular attention include the following:

1. Relationship of dysphagia symptoms to medical treatments (e.g., botulinum toxin injections)
2. Present or past history of unintended weight loss
3. Benefit (or lack thereof) of sensory tricks during meals

4. Rate of eating and drinking
5. Influence of control of the upper extremities, trunk, and head on eating
6. Preferences for liquids vs. solids

As some dystonic conditions may only occur with particular behaviors (i.e., task-specific dystonias), a determination of whether dysphagia is exacerbated or elicited by eating should be attempted.

Clinical Swallow Examination (CSE)

As stated in Chapter 5, the CSE is a powerful tool for swallowing assessment in the hands of a skilled dysphagia clinician. Items deserving of particular attention include:

1. Ability to handle utensils and glassware
2. Pace of eating
3. Posture
4. Use and benefit of sensory tricks
5. Coordination of swallowing and respiration

Videofluoroscopic Swallow Examination (VFSE)

Please see Chapter 6 for general guidelines regarding use of the VFSE. When evaluating individuals with dystonia, areas of particular attention include the following. If possible, approximate the patient's eating posture during the examination and compare swallowing with improved posture. Further explore the effect of sensory tricks on swallowing. Careful attention should be focused on the movement of all structures involved in swallowing, even when those structures are not thought to be involved. Such careful attention is warranted in all cases, but perhaps especially so in patients with dystonia, as it is not uncommon for the distribution of affected musculature to be more widespread than initially thought.

Videoendoscopic Swallow Examination

Chapter 7 provides general guidelines for the use of the videoendoscopic swallow examination. However, little, if any, report of the use of videoendoscopy to evaluate swallowing function in dystonia is available in the literature. The videoendoscopic swallow exam may present with physical challenges for both the patient and the clinician due to the abnormal, twisting postures exhibited in this condition. Additionally, it is known that dystonia is typically exacerbated under stress, and the endoscopic exam may pose a greater challenge in this respect than the VFSE. As with the VFSE, it may be valuable to approximate the patient's eating posture during the exam and compare swallowing with improved posture and explore the effect of sensory tricks on swallowing. During videoendoscopy, careful attention should be focused on the movements of all visible structures involved in swallowing, even when they are not thought to be involved. This procedure may allow the dysphagia clinician to rule out the presence of dystonia in the larynx, pharynx, and velopharynx. Finally, the endoscopic exam may have extra value in patients with laryngeal dystonia (or spasmodic dysphonia) either in isolation and as part of a more distributed dystonia.

Behavioral Management

Dysphagia in individuals with dystonia presents a challenge for behavioral treatment, and there is little data to provide guidance. However, our experience suggests the following observations. When possible, compensatory approaches, particularly postural adjustments, may provide benefit. Sensory tricks such as a light touch to the chin, for example, may also be helpful in providing temporary relief from dystonia. In some patients, this may have a beneficial effect on swallowing. However, it is rare for the patient to have not discovered the benefits of these sensory tricks independently, even though she might not do so consciously or be able to specifically state these benefits. Careful observation is clearly critical during the swallow exam(s).

SUMMARY

Dysphagia is not uncommon to encounter in patients with dystonia when the affected distribution of involved musculature involves the swallowing mechanism. Medical/surgical treatments may be associated with improved, decreased, or unchanged swallowing. Behavioral treatments for dysphagia in those with dystonia present a challenge for even the most skilled clinicians.

19 Ataxia Syndromes

GENERAL DEFINITION

Ataxia is a movement disorder characterized by incoordination in which movement sequences are irregular, incomplete, and erratic. *Undershoot*, in which a movement stops short of target, and *overshoot*, in which a movement goes beyond the target, are frequent descriptors, as is *discoordination* (or dyscoordination). *Dyssynergia* and *dysdiadochokinesis* have also been used as summary descriptors. Holmes (1939) described deficits of rate, range, and force, a division with considerable heuristic appeal. Another way to think about ataxia is provided by Gilman (2004), who observes that in ataxia, muscles that should work together do not. Reduced tone, delayed movement initiation, and intention tremor may also be present in ataxic disorders. In its pure form, ataxia results from cerebellar involvement. The cerebellum plays a major role in coordination of limb, body, and bulbar musculature. Disruption of pathways to and from the cerebellum may also cause ataxia. This general Definition section is one of the longest in this book, because cerebellar abnormalities, especially ataxia, are common in a bewildering number of neurologic diseases and may also result from medical and surgical treatments, such as a relatively rare complication of deep brain stimulation (DBS).

As shown in Table 19-1, Victor and Ropper (2001) include a classification system according to *mode of development and resolution*: acute-transitory, acute-usually reversible, acute-enduring, subacute, and chronic.

The conditions listed under all but the chronic are well known, with the exception perhaps of paraneoplastic. It requires little experience to know that the sound of intoxication is primarily ataxic. Infectious processes that result in inadequate blood supply to the nervous system, as in postanoxic conditions, can also influence the cerebellum or its pathways, as can tumor and multiple sclerosis (MS). In the case of the latter, however, the cerebellum may escape involvement, depending on disease localization, or be part of a more pervasive deficit.

Paraneoplastic syndromes, on the other hand, are patterns of neurologic deficit secondary to cancer of a variety of organs including lung. One mechanism in paraneoplastic syndromes is that of antibodies related to the cancer binding with cells in the nervous system, in this case the cerebellum, thereby disrupting their normal processes. Paslawski, Duffy, and Vernino (2005), as part of

Table 19–1. Classification of disorders characterized partially or exclusively by ataxia

Mode of Development	Selected Etiologies
Acute-transitory	Intoxication
Acute and usually reversible	Post-infectious
Acute-enduring	Postanoxic
Subacute	Brain tumor, paraneoplastic, multiple sclerosis (MS)
Chronic	Friedreich's ataxia (FRDA); olivopontocerebellar degeneration (OPCA) or multiple system atrophy, cerebellar type (MSA-C); cerebellar cortical degeneration

Note. Adapted from *Principles of Neurology* (7th ed., p. 97), by M. Victor and A. H. Ropper, 2001, New York: McGraw-Hill. Reprinted with the permission of the McGraw-Hill Companies.

their analysis of the speech and language of those with paraneoplastic cerebellar syndrome (PCD), found that 12 of 28 patients (43%) reported swallowing difficulty, otherwise unspecified, and one experienced swallowing abnormality as the first sign. Of interest to clinicians is that 10 of the 28 patients (36%) began having cerebellar signs prior to diagnosis of the cancer.

The present chapter will be limited primarily to selected chronic conditions listed in Table 19–1. OPCA, now known primarily as MSA-C, was included with the multiple system atrophies in Chapter 16. The reasons for this selectivity are simple. The acute and transitory or reversible may never come to the swallow clinician's attention or may not need protracted treatment if they do. Dysphagia in acute-enduring and subacute conditions can be recognized generally by the signs described for the chronic conditions (see below), and the treatment of any associated dysphagia in these other conditions such as tumor can also be gleaned from

the treatment suggestions at chapter's end. Nonetheless, the complexity in ataxia syndromes is not yet fully introduced. Another classification system is necessary to fully define the kinds of conditions to be emphasized in this chapter.

Victor and Ropper (2001) further separate the chronic, cerebellar degenerative disorders into three groups: spinocerebellar disorders, which can be further divided into autosomal-recessive and autosomal-dominant forms; cerebellar cortical ataxias; and complex or complicated cerebellar ataxias in which cerebellar signs are mixed with those of other sites of involvement. The lesson in this organization is that ataxia may occur in relative isolation or be accompanied by other neurologic abnormalities. For the dysphagia clinician, these possibilities are important because they prepare them for variety in patient presentation.

The following discussion will emphasize the spinocerebellar atrophies, including Friedreich's ataxia. The other cerebellar atrophies, of which the most frequent is probably MSA-C, have already been described. Because ataxia can occur in almost any neurologic condition, there is no simple way to describe all these conditions. Evaluation and treatment of the spinocerebellar atrophies can be generalized in whole or into other neurologic conditions in which ataxia is a primary influence on swallowing.

ATAXIA SYNDROMES: SPINOCEREBELLAR ATROPHY

Definition

Spinocerebellar atrophy (SCA) is a heterogeneous collection of disorders, most of which begin with involvement of lower limbs and thus gait disturbance (Gilman, 2000). Most are inherited and are generally chronic and progressive. In all, ataxia is a prominent sign, but other systems may also be involved resulting in weakness, abnormal tone, and even myoclonus. Sensory loss including that of position is frequent, and visual and auditory deficits also occur in some types, as does dementia.

The most common form of SCA is *Friedreich's ataxia* (FRDA). FRDA is an autosomal-recessive, inherited disease with some variability in symptoms, but ataxia, reduced reflexes in the legs, upgoing toes, sensory loss, and an early developing dysarthria (and presumably dysphagia) are cardinal signs. The disease may appear in childhood and for a long time was thought to occur only before age 25. Later onset cases, even in the sixth and seventh decades, have now been identified.

Signs and Diagnostic Criteria

According to Victor and Ropper (2001), the earliest sign is nearly always ataxic gait. Ataxia of the upper extremities, and subsequently of the bulbar musculature, is a typical but not inviolate pattern. With involvement of the bulbar musculature both speech and swallowing will likely be impaired. Sensory loss is also a frequent early sign. Tendon reflexes are usually absent. Cardiomyopathy is a frequent non-neurologic sign.

Evolution

Usually, onset is before age 25, but this is not an absolute. Onset may be as early as age 2 and 50% of cases appear before age 10 (Victor & Ropper, 2001). The disease is progressive and bulbar deficits are common after the appearance of limb abnormalities.

Epidemiology

FRDA may be the most common of the inherited ataxia syndromes. The estimated prevalence among Europeans is 1:30,000–50,000 (Victor & Ropper, 2001).

Medical/Surgical Management

FRDA itself seems to be untreatable, but associated conditions such as cardiac abnormalities may respond to traditional medical therapies. Compensatory physical and occupational therapy may be useful. Genetic counseling may be critical.

ATAXIA SYNDROMES: OTHER SPINOCEREBELLAR ATROPHIES

Definition

A variety of autosomal-dominant and autosomal-recessive ataxias also exist (as noted above, FRDA is the most frequent autosomal-recessive form of the disease). Gene research has allowed classification based on genotype (Gilman, 2000). Se-lected autosomal-dominant ataxias, based on genotype, appear in Table 19-2.

A variety of other autosomal-dominant syndromes with predominating ataxic features have been identified. Dentatoru-bropallidoluysian atrophy (DRPLA) is one. Onset may be early (around age 20) or later (onset around age 40). Ataxia may be accompanied by a variety of other movement abnormalities including chorea and myoclonus. Differentiation from Hunting-ton's disease (HD) may be difficult for all but the most experienced examiner.

Table 19–2. Types of autosomal-dominant ataxias with brief descriptions

Type	Description
SCA1	Onset in 30s and 40s typically with ataxia and eventually severe dysarthria and dysphagia secondary to weakness
SCA2	Typical onset in 40s; ataxia, dysarthria, and presumably dysphagia are cardinal features
SCA3, also called Machado-Joseph disease	Onset same as above with ataxia, dysarthria, and dysphagia prominent features; other movement abnormalities also likely
SCA4	May produce a pure cerebellar syndrome
SCA5	May be relatively pure ataxic syndrome with less likelihood of dysphagia
SCA6	May be later onset with episodic appearance of signs
SCA7	Signs similar to other SCAs but includes eventual blindness
SCA8	Characterized by ataxia and bulbar involvement and presumably dysphagia and dysarthria
SCA10	May have complex set of signs including seizures and cognitive impairment; identified only in Mexican population thus far
SCA11	Rare, identified only in the British
SCA12	Begins with tremor and progresses to ataxia and dementia; rare
SCA13–16	All are very rare
SCA17	Very rare; appears to evolve from ataxia to parkinsonism and dementia

Note. Adapted from "The Molecular Genetics of the Ataxia," by G. R. Wilmot and S. H. Subramony, 2004, in R. L. Watts and W. C. Koller (Eds.), *Movement Disorders: Neurologic Principles and Practices* (2nd ed.), New York: McGraw-Hill. Reprinted with the permission of the McGraw-Hill Companies.

Patients with DRPLA may also have seizures, if onset is early, and dementia.

Two types of episodic ataxia are also among the autosomal-dominant syndromes. In EA1, episodes of ataxia are brought on by startle or exercise. EA2 is characterized by longer episodes of ataxia, and stress rather than startle is likely to trigger episodes (Wilmot & Subramony, 2004). To our knowledge, dysphagia has not been described but might be anticipated.

In addition to FRDA, a variety of autosomal-recessive ataxias have also have been identified, as shown in Table 19–3.

Signs/Diagnostic Criteria

Predictably, these conditions are highly variable. Ataxias of body and limbs alone or in combinations are one unifying feature. Ataxia of the bulbar musculature may or may not be present, and when present, may appear early or late. Upper and lower motor neuron involvement, including abnormal tone and weakness, chorea, athetosis, myoclonus, tremor, and dystonia may also occur. Seizures, dementia, and behavioral abnormalities are likely to be present in some as well. Searching for a genetic abnormality is the best way to establish a diagnosis. Clinically, a family history going back as many generations as possible may also be helpful.

Evolution

Age of onset and progression are highly variable. Overall, however, these conditions are degenerative and can be expected in

Table 19–3. The autosomal recessive ataxias	
Disorder	**Description**
Ataxia telangiectasia (AT)	Early onset with multiple telangiectasias and immune system abnormalities in context of progressive neurologic deficits; dysarthria and dysphagia are frequent
Ataxias secondary to vitamin E deficiency	Similar to FRDA
Ataxia with oculomotor apraxia-1	Similar to AT
Autosomal-recessive spastic ataxia of Charlevoix-Saguenay	Rare outside Quebec
Spinocerebellar ataxia with axonal neuropathy	Early onset ataxia
Inborn errors of metabolism	Variable pattern with cognitive impairment in some patients

Note. From "The Molecular Genetics of the Ataxia," by G. R. Wilmot and S. H. Subramony, 2004, in R. L. Watts and W. C. Koller (Eds.), *Movement Disorders: Neurologic Principles and Practices* (2nd ed.), New York: McGraw-Hill. Reprinted with the permission of the McGraw-Hill Companies.

most instances to end in severe disability and death. It may be that the presence of bulbar involvement, especially if dysphagia is present, means a more complicated course, more pulmonary complications, and earlier death. It remains to be seen if alternatives to tube feeding are successful in prolonging life and enhancing quality of life.

Epidemiology

Fortunately, most of these conditions are rare.

Medical Management

Medical management is supportive for the inherited ataxias. For those secondary to a variety of other causes such as vitamin E deficiency, treatment may prevent further degeneration and some improvement may be possible. The poor prognosis for improving ataxia medically is important for the dysphagia expert to recognize. Any improvement in nutrition and hydration will depend upon compensations, although rehabilitation efforts can be justified in some instances, as will be discussed below.

SWALLOWING IN ATAXIA

Epidemiology

Although the cerebellum is part of a distributed network supporting swallowing (Harris et al., 2005; Suzuki et al., 2003), the presence of ataxia does not guarantee the presence of dysphagia. In some conditions, the bulbar musculature may be spared, and in some even ataxia of the bulbar musculature fails to produce a dysphagia of functional significance (i.e., impacting safety, adequacy, or pleasure). Nonetheless, in some conditions dysphagia is likely. OPCA or what is increasingly being called MSA-C (see Chapter 16) may be the cerebellar syndrome with the highest incidence of dysphagia, being 72% in OPCA and 38% in a small sample of "unexplained" adult-onset cases of ataxia (Abele et al., 2002). Descriptions of the dysphagia were not provided.

Jardim and colleagues (2001) report that 30 of 47 (64%) patients with Machado-Joseph disease (SCA-3) had dysphagia and that it appears later in this disease. Nagaya and colleagues (2004) report aspiration in 30% of a group of patients with what they call "degenerative cerebellar ataxia." This percent was derived from videofluoroscopic examination, making the number somewhat more convincing. It is to be remembered, of course, that one can be significantly dysphagic without aspirating. Had all signs of dysphagia been included, the percent might have been higher.

In some of the autosomal-dominant ataxia syndromes such as SCA-1, the presence of life-threatening dysphagia in the disease's latter stage appears nearly inevitable. Victor and Ropper (2001) also identify dysphagia as a nearly inevitable late stage sign in FRDA and as a significant threat to life.

A possible way for the clinician to consider the presence and importance of dysphagia in cerebellar disease is to consider two variables:

1. Whether the condition is limited to the cerebellum or has extended to

other portions of the sensorimotor and cognitive networks in support of bulbar functions

2. Duration of the condition

The greater the extent of involvement and the longer the duration, the more likely it is that the person will have a functionally significant dysphagia.

Symptoms

We have seen a variety of patients with ataxia alone and in combination with other deficits. In general, the more extensive the deficit, the longer the symptom list, although some may not admit to dysphagia even if they have had choking episodes (Nilsson, Ekberg, Olsson, & Hindfelt, 1996). A careful history usually is sufficient to uncover symptoms, however. When the syndrome is purely ataxic, symptom variability and relative mildness is the norm, although in severe ataxia, severe symptoms may be reported. What follows is a summary of our clinical experience, beginning with those symptoms we associate with relatively pure cerebellar involvement leading primarily to incoordination.

1. Variable choking and coughing, most severe when tired, distracted, or with especially challenging boluses
2. Slowness of bolus preparation
3. Variable occurrence of a sticking sensation
4. Variable difficulty managing saliva
5. Greater difficulty on liquids than solids (Ramio-Torrenta, Gomez, & Genis, 2006)
6. Excessive time to eat
7. Fatigue during meals

8. Nasopharyngeal reflux (i.e., material exiting through the nose)

Of course, all other symptoms are possible as well, although their occurrence is usually variable. As weakness, abnormal tone, and other movement abnormalities occur, the usual effect is to make these symptoms more frequent and more severe.

Signs

Underdiagnosis of dysphagia in ataxia syndromes is being changed by the increasing reliance upon instrumental swallowing examinations. The following signs may be encountered.

Oral Stage

Signs of oral stage abnormality (FRDA in two cases, autosomal-dominant, otherwise unspecified in five, and unknown in one case) can be absent (Nilsson et al., 1996). Others report:

1. Oral residual
2. Coating of the hard palate in some patients
3. Less commonly, late velar elevation
4. Premature spillage occurring at approximately the same frequency as delayed velar elevation (Ramio-Torrenta et al., 2006)

Pharyngeal Stage

In those same patients, six of eight (75%) had pharyngeal abnormalities including:

1. Reduced epiglottic inversion
2. Coating on the posterior pharyngeal wall

3. Delayed initiation of the pharyngeal stage of swallowing
4. Residue in the valleculae and pyriform sinuses
5. Impaired upper esophageal sphincter (UES) relaxation (Ramio-Torrenta et al, 2006)

Laryngeal Stage

1. Penetration
2. Aspiration
3. Both perhaps more frequent with extension of disease outside the cerebellum and especially into the brainstem

Functional Consequences

No data on functional consequences are known to us, but knowing the signs allows one to speculate. Ataxia of the limbs alone or in combination with weakness and abnormal tone may make eating difficult. Unpredictable ability to move food and liquid into the mouth may also disrupt oral stage preparation and movement of the bolus, with subsequent difficulties during the pharyngeal stage. As a result, eating and drinking may be inefficient, unpleasant, and risky. Similar results may occur because of incoordination of oral, pharyngeal, and laryngeal events. Even in the absence of risk, pleasure may drain from the rituals of eating and drinking. Eating and drinking may become unpredictable and untidy adventures that force the person to avoid eating or drinking in front of others.

Health Consequences

As disease duration increases, pulmonary consequences in some ataxia syndromes appear more likely. Respiratory complications were the most common causes of death in one study of patients with SCA1 (Genis et al., 1995). Poor nutritional status including weight and weight/height ratios in those with dysphagia have been identified (Lefton-Greif et al., 2000). Swallowing and nutritional parameters probably exist as a complex interaction. Life-threatening or fatal choking may occur.

Evaluation

Chapters 4, 5, 6, and 7 contain detail of the generic evaluation procedures. In this section only the special features of evaluation in ataxia syndromes are highlighted.

Chart Review and History

Because the ataxia syndromes are so variable and often complex, the chart review and history are likely to take longer than in some of the more straightforward conditions such as Parkinson's disease (PD). Of special interest are the following.

Medical Diagnosis. This is critical because of the variability in the likelihood of dysphagia during the disease's course. For example, Burk and colleagues (1996) identified dysphagia in 89% of those with SCA1, 54% in those with SCA2, and 34% in those with SCA3.

Duration of Illness. Dysphagia may occur early or late, more frequently late, but the clinician should have a high degree of suspicion that potentially significant dysphagia may be evolving prior to its easy recognition by medical providers and even family and patient. It may be that early identification can lead to interventions to slow dysphagia's development or prevent its health consequences. In addition, early onset may sometimes be associated with more rapid decline, in contrast to some cases of MSA in which later onset may presage more rapid decline (Klockgether et al., 1998).

Degree of Impairment. In some ataxia syndromes, the degree of impairment, whether the patient is ambulatory or bedridden, whether able to feed self or not, may be a better predictor of dysphagia than is duration of disease (Jardim et al., 2001).

Spread of Disease. Retrieving information on the full array of each patient's signs and presumed sites of involvement is also critical in dysphagia. It appears that dysphagia is more likely and more severe as disease extends into the brainstem (Rub et al., 2003).

Symptoms of Dysphagia. Symptoms of dysphagia and who identified these (i.e., patient, family, or health care provider) are useful.

Sensory Loss. Varying severities of hearing and vision loss, in addition to proprioceptive and other sensory changes, may occur (David et al, 1998). Sensory loss of all sorts may impact patient performance and complicate both evaluation and treatment.

Clinical Swallow Examination (CSE)

The variability of swallowing impairments in this population makes a careful CSE especially critical. The CSE allows many more swallows under realistic conditions than are possible with instrumental examination. If time permits, the following may be informative:

1. Examination of the bulbar structures (i.e., lips, jaw, tongue, palate, and larynx) and the respiratory mechanism for signs of incoordination, weakness, and abnormal tone. Follow the guidelines in Chapter 5. This examination will support hypotheses about whether the disease is confined to the cerebellum or has extended into brainstem, basal ganglia, and cortex.

2. To the degree training and the environment permit, test each individual's ability to cut up food, load a fork or spoon, and move food into the mouth. If possible, let each person do this without help. Both independent ability and what assistance is required, such as cutting up meat, loading the fork, cueing about bite size, and so on, should be noted.

3. Observe each individual's ability to drink from glass, cup, and straw. Again, note what assistance, if any, is required.

4. Take special note of any conditions that seem to accompany and perhaps cause choking or other threats to pleasurable, sufficient, and safe eating and drinking.

Videofluoroscopic Swallow Examination (VFSE)

Chapter 6 contains a complete description of the videofluoroscopic swallow examination (VFSE). That chapter prepares the clinician for most movement disordered dysphagia patients. Ataxia, however, because of the potential prominence of incoordination in both limbs and swallowing structures, may require some special attention. It is recommended that the following considerations be included.

Allow patient-controlled boluses on spoon and from cup. Doing so will highlight ataxic difficulties of the limbs that may complicate oropharyngeal swallowing. Use challenging boluses such as barium paste and large, solid boluses of real food. The incoordination may be less obvious unless such boluses are used during the examination. Be sure to read the exam repeatedly as incoordination as a cause of residue or penetration-aspiration may only be obvious from repeated viewing of a swallow with an eye toward systematically observing different structures and bolus interactions on multiple viewing.

Videoendoscopic Swallow Evaluation

Chapter 7 details the videoendoscopic swallow examination. We generally prefer VFSE for instrumental assessment of swallowing in patients with ataxia as a prominent sign, as we find the coordination of oropharyngeal swallowing events is best visualized via VFSE. Of course, exceptions exist to every rule and indications for videoendoscopy are provided in the appropriate section of Chapter 7. We know of little report of the use of videoendoscopy to evaluate swallowing function in patients with ataxia in the literature, but as with the VFSE, patient-controlled boluses on spoon and from cup may be valuable to highlight ataxic difficulties of the limbs that may complicate the swallow seems sensible. Multiple readings of the exam are also of critical importance as incoordination as a cause of dysphagia may likely only be obvious

with close observation of the different structures and bolus interactions upon multiple viewings.

Treatment

Medical

As Paulson and Ammache (2001) observed, evaluation has outstripped treatment for ataxia disorders (as in many other conditions). They recommend that every person with an episodic ataxia be given a trial of acetazolamide and that any accompanying spasticity be treated medically. Some other signs such as seizures can also be treated with traditional medical approaches. Those authors identify physical therapy and speech therapy for swallowing dysfunction as being "particularly useful" (p. 779). In other words, swallowing evaluation and treatment are likely to be foremost among the therapeutic options. It is important to remember that interventions for some signs associated with ataxia (like dystonia) such as botulinum toxin for oropharyngeal dystonia can cause dysphagia (Tuite & Lang, 1996).

Surgical

No surgical treatments are routinely available for treatment of ataxia.

Behavioral Therapy

Compensations are most frequently the general approach of greatest potential benefit, especially if cerebellar involvement is relatively pure. If weakness and reduced tone are also part of the pathophysiology, then a variety of the rehabilitative methods may also be appropriate:

Chapters 13 and 14 describe compensatory and rehabilitation techniques approaches in depth. In this section we merely highlight those methods likely to be of greatest benefit.

Compensatory Approaches. All compensations to improve safety and efficiency can be tried. The risk is that thickeners, alternative food preparations, and even postures can threaten perceived quality of life. Therefore, it is critical that evaluation convincingly demonstrate that prandial aspiration is a threat to the patient's health and that postures do indeed improve safety and/or efficiency. In the absence of that proof (or strong suspicion), it may be better to do nothing beyond counseling and the offering of systematic follow-up. Compensations in posture that may help prevent having to change liquid and food preparation are:

1. Chin tuck (Nagaya, Kachi, Yamada, & Sumi, 2004). However, this method should never be reflexively tried, as aspiration from the pyriform sinuses may be made more likely and control of the bolus in the mouth more difficult.
2. Head stabilization: Our most frequent postural adjustment is to look for methods for stabilizing the patient's head. Resting the head against a high-backed chair or against the wall prior to swallowing may be accompanied by increased safety and efficiency without posing a significant threat to pleasure.
3. Weighted equipment: Weighted plates and utensils may help to control ataxia and increase efficiency of eating.
4. Special drinking cups: Cups to control the amount of bolus available on

each sip and to prevent liquid from sloshing out may make drinking more efficient and pleasurable.

Rehabilitation Techniques. The method(s) of rehabilitation depends on whether ataxia alone or in combination with strength and tone abnormalities predominates. Ataxia can be seen as a loss of skill. Therefore, it makes sense to try increasing swallowing skill. Probably, simply urging the patient to swallow more carefully will not be effective, because most patients, in our experience, try to do just that on their own. Therefore, intensive skill training, especially if other neuropathologies such as weakness are relatively minor, may be helpful, especially if combined with head stabilization. We recommend consideration of one or more of the effortful swallowing variations, including the Showa maneuver (see p. 103). If aspiration results from ataxia, then the supraglottic swallow can be employed (see p. 99). If significant residue remains in the valleculae postswallow, employ the Mendelsohn maneuver (if cognition allows; see p. 94) or head raise exercise (if a simpler exercise is indicated; see p. 97).

If ataxia is present along with strength or tone abnormality, depending on how it is distributed, one or more of the strengthening exercises may be helpful. Consider the following alone or in combinations:

1. Lingual strengthening (see p. 88) if tongue abnormality is a major contributor and if the equipment is available. If not, strengthening with tongue blades, done properly, is a reasonable approach.
2. RMST (see p. 83) if respiratory deficits predominate.

3. LSVT (see p. 81) if general weakness or hypotonia appears as a major explanation for the dysphagia.

4. Masako maneuver (see p. 101), again if tongue or pharyngeal weakness appears prominent and if tongue strengthening equipment is unavailable.

5. Electrical stimulation (see p. 108) if it appears to help during VFSE, which is now highly recommended as a first step in considering this approach in any of its various forms, especially electrical stimulation over the neck.

SUMMARY

The ataxia syndromes are many and varied. The clinician's first obligation is to recognize as many of these syndromes as possible. Doing so will inform about the medical context in which management will subsequently take place. The second and more critical obligation is careful assessment and appropriate treatment planning and execution.

20 Chorea

CHOREA

Definition

Chorea is the name for a typically complex set of quick, irregular, and jerky abnormal movements. Choreatic movements may involve only one or a limited number of body structures with the usual pattern, especially as the condition worsens, of combined trunk and body part involvement. Dystonia and athetosis, two other patterns of movement abnormality, are often difficult to distinguish from chorea, and some patients may have two or even all three of these movement patterns. Nonetheless, traditional neurology attempts to distinguish them and other abnormal movement patterns, a tradition to be carried on in this volume. Therefore, choreatic movements are to be distinguished from the slower, writhing movements of *athetosis*; the quicker, often more regular, and generally less widely distributed abnormal movement patterns called *myoclonus*; the more sustained abnormal movements called *dystonia*; and the more regular, often stereotyped movement abnormality called *dyskinesia*. It is to be recalled that chorea is a sign and not a disease, although it has been folded into the name of a limited number of diseases, notably *Huntington's chorea* (more commonly known now as *Huntington's disease* [HD]) and *Sydenham's chorea* (SC).

SC develops in some children after an infectious process and in the majority of cases spontaneously resolves over months. Its prevalence in the United States is much reduced given advances in antibiotic therapy. If it does occur and persists, medical and behavioral management of the type described below for the treatment of HD may be warranted.

A number of other conditions presenting with chorea, listed below, may come to the clinician's attention. Management of dysphagia in these other conditions may be patterned after that suggested for HD, the condition whose characteristics and management form the bulk of this chapter. These other conditions include the following.

Chorea Gravidarum

Pregnancy is an infrequent cause of chorea, as is the use of oral contraceptives, and is called chorea gravidarum. It usually resolves spontaneously after delivery or when contraceptives are discontinued.

173

Systemic Lupus Erythematosus

Systemic lupus erythematosus (SLE) is characterized by chronic inflammation secondary to an autoimmune response that can attack the body's organs, including the brain. One manifestation of nervous system involvement is chorea. A related condition is primary antiphospholipid antibody syndrome (PAPS).

Wilson's Disease

See Chapter 23.

Dentatorubropallidoluysian Atrophy

Dentatorubropallidoluysian atrophy (DRPLA) is an inherited condition characterized by cell loss in the dentate and red nuclei, the globus pallidus, and the subthalamic nucleus. Signs may be highly variable, but chorea is one possible presentation.

Acanthocytosis

Acanthocytosis with chorea is a rare, inherited condition beginning in late childhood or early adulthood and characterized by chorea and dementia, although tics, dystonia, and rigidity can also appear. If dystonia is present, it is likely to be an action dystonia involving the tongue (Mark, 2004). Oral stage abnormalities would be expected. The chorea, which usually predominates, may begin in the bulbar musculature and represent another reason for dysphagia perhaps of both oral and pharyngeal stages. A related condition is McLeod's disease, also a rare,

inherited disease. Onset is in middle age or later. According to Ropper and Brown (2005), facial involvement is less frequent than in other diseases causing chorea, and therefore dysphagia should be less likely.

Senile Chorea

Senile chorea is a controversial diagnosis. Those who believe in it advocate for differentiating it from HD and report that it begins later than Huntington's and in the absence of a family history.

Vascular Chorea

Vascular chorea has acute onset resulting from stroke. Recovery is often relatively rapid. Predictably, the chorea is usually confined to one side of the body.

Other Causes

Other causes of chorea include metabolic disorders such as hyperthyroidism and hypocalcemia. In addition medications such as neuroleptics, substances such as cocaine, systemic diseases such as AIDS, stroke, tumor, infectious processes, and toxins are among the additional potential causes of chorea (Mark, 2001).

HUNTINGTON'S DISEASE (HD)

Definition

HD is an inherited neurodegenerative condition characterized by chorea (usually beginning in the hands and face), behavior change, and dementia. Its relentless advance ends in profound dementia, anarthria, aphagia, and death. Average duration of disease is approximately 15–20 years.

A genetic abnormality, now identifiable with a blood test, is by far the most frequent cause of HD. Brain imaging confirms bilateral involvement of the head of caudate and putamen. Frontal and temporal lobe atrophy may also be identified during the course of the disease.

Signs/Diagnostic Criteria

Behavior, cognition, and movement all change in reasonably predictable ways. Behavior changes include distractibility, irritability, argumentativeness, and becoming withdrawn. Intellectual decline may include poor problem solving and confusion. Interestingly, memory is often preserved until late in the disease's course. The movement abnormality usually appears first in the extremities and face, and early on a person may be described simply as restless or fidgety. The appearance of the behavioral and cognitive changes may be simultaneous or variable, and they may occur before, after, or at the same time as the movement abnormality. It may well be that the later the disease onset, the more likely that behavior and cognitive decline will occur after, sometimes well after, the motor deterioration begins. Whereas the movement abnormality may be delayed in those with earlier onset, motor change may be the predominant sign in those with late-onset dementia. In our experience, even when general cognition seems relatively well preserved, decreased initiation of activity becomes an increasingly significant sign, and one with no small consequence for family and other caregivers.

For example, if asked, family members may well report that the person is increasingly unlikely to initiate conversation.

Motor signs may be somewhat variable, and patients may be differentiated by their general motor signs. For example, Kagel and Leopold (1992) distinguished what they called hyperkinetic patients from those in whom rigidity and bradykinesia predominated. The rigid predominant form of the disease is sometimes called the *Westphal variant*. In addition, signs may evolve over time, with dystonia and rigidity dominating the chorea as the disease progresses. Similarly, the behavioral signs may change, with early irritability and later apathy as but one example.

Any combination of behavioral and cognitive decline with choreatic movements in a person with a family history of HD strongly suggests the diagnosis. This clinical diagnosis can be confirmed with a DNA evaluation.

A variety of scales have been developed to support quantification of assessment in HD. Typical of those is the *Unified Huntington's Disease Rating Scale* (UHDRS; Huntington Study Group, 1996). This scale is actually a collection of scales and questionnaires that allow sampling of motor impairment, cognitive ability, and behavior, as well as functional abilities. Users of this tool (Klempir, Klemfirova, Spackova, Zidovska, & Roth, 2006) have noted the absence of nutrition and swallowing scales or questions and recommend that both be systematically evaluated using standardized tools.

The motor part of the UHDRS samples chorea, eye signs, dystonia, parkinsonian signs such as rigidity, gait, and bulbar functions. The bulbar functions that are specifically assessed are dysarthria and tongue protrusion, presumably because of the tradition of having persons with neurologic disease protrude their tongues as part of the neurologic examination.

Evolution

The behavioral abnormality may evolve into serious psychosis. In addition, the patient is likely to descend into severe dementia and be incapable of initiating or responding. The movement abnormality may become more complex, especially the dystonia and chorea, and also more widely distributed across body structures. Flailing movements may become more severe, so that the patient has trouble staying seated, and facial distortion, tongue protrusion, and grunting may all signal the disease's advance. Of special concern to the swallowing clinician is the fact that for many, impaired nutritional status and weight loss increase as the disease progresses, and body weight may be a predictor of disease course (Trejo, Boll, Alonso, Ochoa, & Velasquez, 2005). Unless patients die from another cause, they are likely to end up institutionalized and requiring total care. Death typically occurs after 15 to 20 years but may come sooner. In late stage disease, patients with HD are typically *anarthric* (speechless), *aphagic* (unable to swallow), demented, and totally dependent.

Epidemiology

HD occurs in approximately 4 of every million persons, but the rate seems to be higher in those of Northern European descent. HD can appear in childhood but most frequently starts in the 40s or 50s, though it can appear later. Males and females appear equally likely to inherit the disease (Marshall, 2004).

Medical/Surgical Management

HD cannot be cured, and no surgical approach is of known benefit for the chorea, although botulinum toxin injections may relieve dystonia. Bonelli, Wenning, and Kapfhammer (2004) have surveyed the double-blind randomized trials of medical treatments and make the following recommendations:

1. Delay medical treatment during the disease's early stage.
2. If medications have been tried, discontinue them to see the effect on movement and other functions.
3. When treatment is appropriate, they suggest a variety of medications including haloperidol, although at the smallest possible dosage, as high dosages may cause a number of complications including worsening dysphagia.
4. Depression may respond to selective serotonin reuptake inhibitors.
5. Atypical antipsychotic medications may reduce behavioral abnormalities.
6. Psychotherapy and physical, occupational, and speech therapy are recommended.
7. Genetic testing and family counseling are also recommended.

SWALLOWING IN HUNTINGTON'S DISEASE

Epidemiology

Eating and swallowing abnormalities occur in nearly 100% of patients with HD. Irregular, unpredictable, rapid movements of the limbs, body, face, tongue, larynx, pharynx, velum, and respiratory mechanism are the primary explanation. Early on, if behavior and mentation are relatively intact, signs of dysphagia may be extremely variable even in the same person. This variability seems to result from irregular breakdowns in the intricate coordination swallowing requires as abnormal movements flash about the swallowing structures. For example, if a sudden uncontrolled inhalation occurs as a bolus is passing into the pharynx, that bolus may be sucked into the larynx and trachea. If movement suddenly invades the tongue, the bolus may move unexpectedly into the pharynx in the absence of the usual sequence of pharyngeal and laryngeal events that guarantee a normal swallow. Yorkston, Miller, & Strand (2004) report more specifically on the occurrence of other swallow-related abnormalities. They observe that respiratory deficit secondary to chorea of the respiratory muscles occurs in 40% of patients. They cite a frequency of 10% for aspiration and *aerophagia* (swallowing of air), and 40% for *eructation* or excessive belching. As in other movement disorders, complications of dysphagia can contribute to morbidity and mortality.

Symptoms

The full range of symptoms may be reported, although caregivers are much more likely to describe symptoms than patients are to report them. Symptoms of *tachyphagia* or rapid eating are frequently reported by family. Also frequent are reports of coughing and choking. Dependence for eating is nearly inevitable. "Messy" eating, with difficulty getting food and drink to the mouth, if a patient continues to self-feed is also a common complaint. It is also common that food falls from the mouth.

Signs

Kagel & Leopold (1992) summarize 16 years of evaluating dysphagia in HD. The following main features are derived primarily from their report of systematic clinical and videofluoroscopic examinations. Because of the complexity of abnormal movements in chorea, the division into oral and pharyngeal stages and aspiration-penetration does not work perfectly. Therefore, signs are combined in this section.

In those with primary rigidity, mandibular rigidity leads to slower bolus preparation. Other signs include prolonged oral transit; oral residuals; incoordination of the oral and pharyngeal stages of swallowing, with uncontrolled spillage of the bolus into the pharynx; disrupted coordination of swallowing and respiration with inappropriately timed inhalations during pharyngeal transit (more common in those with chorea predominating over rigidity); long delays in swallow initiation; audible inspirations, sniffing, and grunting reflecting respiratory chorea, which may also disrupt coordination of swallowing and respiration; "abrupt, audible swallows" (p. 108); and penetration and aspiration.

In the report of one carefully studied case, Hamakawa and colleagues (2004) add additional details, including:

1. Reduced anterior movement of the hyoid upon swallow.
2. Reduced inversion of the epiglottis upon swallow.

3. Reduced motion of the tongue back to the posterior pharyngeal wall upon swallow initiation.
4. UES opening at the borderland of normal duration.

Our own observations confirm the above findings, to which we would add:

1. Near pathologically fast pharyngeal stage
2. Reduced extent and duration of UES opening
3. Poor airway protection during the swallow
4. Prolonged chewing of solid and even some semisolid boluses
5. Variably adequate lip seal leading to escape of the bolus anteriorly

Tube feeding may be required if hydration and nutrition parameters cannot be maintained or if choking and pneumonia are frequent. Of course, tube feeding presents some ethical dilemmas depending on the patient's and family's wishes.

Functional/Quality of Life Influences

We could find no data. However, the impression from our own practice is that the impact of the dysphagia is felt much more acutely by the family than by the patient. Probably, the quality of life impact from the swallowing problem is dwarfed by the impact of the chorea and other potential movement abnormalities. Children may feel the additional anguish of knowing the disease can be inherited, as may parents who recognize their genetic contribution to the condition.

Health Consequences

The full range of health consequences is possible, and special attention should be given to weight loss and decreased body mass index; whether these are due to increased energy requirements, difficulty with eating and swallowing, or as another manifestation of the disease process is debated (Trejo et al., 2004). Other consequences include:

1. Malnutrition and dehydration
2. Dependence for nutrition
3. Death by asphyxia from solid food aspiration
4. Pneumonia

Swallowing Evaluation

Chart Review and History

The chart review and history are discussed in Chapter 4. Most of what a clinician wants to discover is discussed there. Recall that the family is likely to be a better source of information than the patient, depending on duration of cognitive, behavioral, and motor signs. However, in HD and other conditions causing chorea, special emphasis can be placed on:

1. Date of onset and signs at onset
2. Eating habits, looking for tachyphagia and behavioral and cognitive threats to normal hydration and nutrition
3. Other behavioral abnormalities
4. Signs of dementia
5. Duration and type of movement abnormalities
6. Family history of the disease, including outcome

7. Presence/absence of family and genetic counseling
8. Involvement of other family members, given the disease is inherited and behavioral problems may predominate
9. History of medical management and plans for future treatments
10. Health consequences of swallowing
11. Results of nutritional evaluation and plans for nutritional management
12. Evidence of declining interest and participation
13. Any history of swallowing abnormality
14. Evidence of dependence for activities of daily living, including feeding oneself
15. History of previous health or quality of life consequences of eating or swallowing abnormality

Clinical Swallow Examination (CSE

The clinical swallow examination (CSE) can be especially important in chorea because of the behavioral and cognitive complications for swallowing that may compound the motor deficit. The goals are to document the distribution of chorea across the bulbar and respiratory structures and complete an eating examination to document possible tachyphagia and other behavioral abnormalities. In addition to the usual procedures as described in Chapter 5, the following may be helpful.

To get an estimate of respiratory chorea, have patient hold breath and inhale and exhale slowly and as evenly as possible. Teasing out the presence of laryngeal chorea may not be easy, but observing the difference in performance on simple breathing and on vowel prolongation while observing respiration and then movement of larynx in the neck may help. Palpation and visualization of the external portions of the respiratory mechanism may be valuable.

Simple observation of lips, rest of face, tongue, and palate at rest and during maximum performance testing and with speech should be adequate to establish distribution of chorea.

An eating examination done as naturalistically as possible may well reveal tachyphagia and its possible relationship to coughing and choking. It may also reveal breakdowns in the coordination of swallowing and respiration as evidenced by, for example, abrupt inhalations while swallowing.

Videofluoroscopic Swallow Examination (VFSE)

Procedures for the videofluoroscopic swallow examination (VFSE) are discussed in Chapter 6. In chorea, several procedures may be of special importance:

1. Observation of structures at rest in both lateral and anterior-posterior (AP) views and of course during all bolus swallows.
2. Contrasting clinician- and self-administered boluses of normal (15 to 20 mL) size.
3. Testing with and without a variety of postural compensations. The compensations are listed below in the compensatory treatment section.
4. Testing with any special utensils—cups, straws, and so on—the patient uses at home.

Videoendoscopic Swallow Examination

The complete endoscopic examination is described in Chapter 7.

Behavioral Treatment

Bilney, Morris, and Perry (2003) observe on the basis of a review of the treatment literature that there is "a small amount of evidence to support the use of speech pathology for the management of eating and swallowing disorders" (p. 12). A small amount is better than none, but clearly much more work must be done. Nonetheless, swallowing therapy is often recommended, but no data on effect of rehabilitative and only limited data on compensatory approaches appear to have been published. The following section on compensations is largely derived from the work of Kagel and Leopold (1992). The section on rehabilitation is based on speculation arising from our clinical practice.

Compensatory Approaches

Data from Kagel and Leopold (1992) support the following compensations:

1. A wedge to reduce hyperextension, if present
2. Slight chin tuck posture
3. Slight trunk flexion
4. Positioning tray of food at or below waist level
5. Preceding regular boluses with lemon ice bolus
6. Weighted cup
7. Wrist weights
8. Leg weights
9. Nonskid mats
10. Scoop dishes
11. Reduced bowl and utensil size

These compensations work for those of mild to moderate severity and are worth trying later in the disease, though they are less likely to be of substantive benefit. Kagel and Leopold (2003) reported that selected items of these compensations combined with Valsalva's maneuver (forcible laryngeal valving) allowed 11 of 12 patients (92%) to return to normal diets.

Rehabilitation Techniques

If a patient has significant dementia, any rehabilitation is likely to be unsuccessful and merely compound behavioral problems. If mentation is reasonably intact and if patient shows some insight into presence of dysphagia, a rehabilitative program could be recommended. By the time significant dysphagia appears it is likely that behavior and cognition will have declined as well. However, depending on the pattern of difficulty, the following simple exercises may make sense:

1. Hard or effortful swallow (see p. 104)
2. Showa maneuver (see p. 103)
3. LSVT (see p. 81)
4. Intention treatment (see p. 106)

When behavioral approaches are unsuccessful, tube feeding may need to be offered to those with severe weight loss or other swallowing-related complications. The issue is very complex, however. It is worth remembering that aspirators will aspirate. Less controversial is the use of dietary supplements. Supplementation is considered an imperative by Trejo and colleagues (2005). Such supplementation may prolong patient life. It may even help to retard the nearly inevitable decline in swallowing competence.

SUMMARY

Chorea can manifest itself in a variety of conditions, most commonly HD. Dysphagia can be expected to occur when choreatic movements occur in the swallowing mechanism and be exacerbated by behavioral and intellectual decline. Long-term involvement with a dysphagia clinician is important, especially considering that patients with HD, for example, may survive for 15 to 20 years after onset.

21 Dyskinesia

DYSKINESIA

Definition

For some, dyskinesia is a class of movement disorders that includes tremor, chorea, and dystonia. For others, dyskinesia deserves its own place among the movement abnormalities. We have adopted the latter position, primarily for pedagogic reasons. This position requires that we mention the frequency with which dyskinesia appears with other movement disorders such as dystonia and Parkinson's disease (PD). Considered as a separate abnormality, an operational definition of dyskinesia is that of *a moderately fast, repetitive, frequent (although this may vary), and often stereotypic movement*. Of concern to dysphagia clinicians, dyskinesia can involve the limbs, trunk, head, oral, pharyngeal, and laryngeal structures, alone or in combinations.

Dyskinesia is most frequently diagnosed as a side effect of medical management of PD and as tardive dyskinesia (TD) most commonly associated with the phenothiazines, a class of antipsychotic neuroleptic drugs used to treat severe mental illness such as schizophrenia and mania. In PD, drug-induced dyskinesia is usually treated with medical and surgical approaches. For example, some medications may have a positive influence on levodopa-induced dyskinesia, such as MAO-B inhibitors, COMT inhibitors, amantadine, and dopamine agonists (Jankovic & Stacy, 2007). Surgical intervention (e.g., deep brain stimulation [DBS]) may also be considered, and dyskinesia following prolonged levodopa therapy is a common indication for this approach. Interestingly, in one study, PD patients with dyskinesia had superior swallowing to those without, a phenomenon the authors attribute to increased levodopa dosage (Monte, da Silva-Junior, Brag-Neto, Nobre e Souza, & de Bruin, 2005). Haloperidol, an antipsychotic drug pharmacologically related to the phenothiazines, is the usual medication implicated in the onset of TD. The atypical neuroleptic olanzapine appears to have reduced the occurrence of TD (Caroff, Mann, Campbell, & Sullivan, 2002). Indeed, the presence of TD sufficient to alter swallowing would seem to be relatively rare, at least in the United States, depending on the sophistication of medical management. If psychiatrically feasible, ideal management of TD is the immediate discontinuation of the associated medication. Psychiatric reevaluation to consider alternative diagnoses and treatments may be valuable. If antipsychotic medications are required to control psychiatric disease, atypical neuroleptics should be considered (Tarsy, 2000). Clearly, physicians are strongly motivated to provide treatment because of the severity of the psychiatric problems in many cases, even when the drugs have negative consequences such as TD. TD has received considerable research attention, despite its apparent reduced incidence due to new classes of medication. The next section is devoted primarily to TD.

TARDIVE DYSKINESIA

Definition

Tardive dyskinesia (TD) is a reasonably stereotyped pattern of abnormal movements often involving only the face and tongue, although other bulbar structures can be involved. In some instances, rather than stereotypic, movements may be irregular and unpredictable. The cause is the neuroleptic management of severe mental illness, usually with use of phenothiazines. It was once called "fly-catcher tongue" because of the frequent quick tongue protrusions and retractions that are seen in many patients (Friedman, 1998). Other forms of tardive movement are described by Goetz and Horn (2004), including tardive tremor, tardive akathisia, and tardive dystonia. The implication of these terms is that neuroleptics can cause tremor, a sense of restlessness, and dystonia. Less commonly, TD can be induced by other medications (Friedman, 1998).

Signs/Diagnostic Criteria

Abnormal movements, often stereotypes of the face and tongue caused by the use of antipsychotic medications that often persist after a drug is withdrawn, are the main signs. As Ropper and Brown (2005) say, "tardive dyskinesia has come to refer to striking, repetitive, stereotyped, almost rhythmic mouth and tongue movements" (p. 95). Relationship to medications is the key criterion. Movements can also involve the pharynx, larynx, respiratory mechanism, trunk, and extremities.

Evolution

TD can worsen with prolonged use of antipsychotic medications but may disappear if the medication is stopped at the first appearance of the movement abnormality. However, TD may persist after the discontinuation of the medication. Cases of resolution despite continued medical treatment have also been reported, and occasionally symptoms may even worsen after drug withdrawal. Dyskinesia in other conditions such as PD can be expected to increase in severity with disease duration and exposure to levodopa. With prolonged use of antipsychotic medications, a potentially fatal condition called *neuroleptic malignant syndrome* (NMS) can occur. The most common signs of this syndrome are fever, increasingly severe rigidity, and mental status changes, often beginning with drowsiness progressing to coma. This condition requires quick recognition and treatment (Ropper & Brown, 2005).

Epidemiology

Historical data suggest that with traditional neuroleptics, 5% to 45% of hospitalized psychiatric patients develop TD compared to approximately 30% of outpatients. Dyskinesia can also develop in persons not on such medications, but this is a relatively rare occurrence. TD may be more likely in women than men. Dyskinesia in PD is induced by prolonged levodopa use (Fernandez, Rodriguez, Skidmore, & Okun, 2007).

Medical/Surgical Management

Medical Management

Tarsy (2000) provides some guidelines for medical management of TD associated with neuroleptics. If the psychiatric condition allows, immediate discontinuation of the medication should be completed. Psychiatric reevaluation should be completed to reassess diagnosis and treatment. If antipsychotic medications are necessary, atypical neuroleptics should be considered, which are associated with a reduced risk of developing this condition (Caroff et al., 2002).

Botulinum toxin injections may be of value. For example, Feve and colleagues (1993) report the positive effects of botulinum toxin to treat laryngeal dyskinesia affecting respiration. The feeling of shortness of breath both during rest and exercise was reduced.

Surgical Management

DBS is the surgical treatment for patients with PD and levodopa-induced dyskinesia. DBS of the globus pallidus internus (GPi) has been established to reduce dyskinesia quite dramatically, with an approximate 75% decrease in dyskinesia scores following surgery (The Deep Brain Stimulation for Parkinson's Disease Study Group [DBSPDSG], 2001; Krack et al., 2003; Volkman et al., 1998). Three years after surgery, a 50% reduction in dyskinesia scores has been reported (Durif, Lemaire, Debilly, & Dordian, 2002).

The influence on dyskinesia associated with surgery appears to be independent of medication dose changes as GPi DBS does not usually result in reduction of dopaminergic medications (DBSPDSG, 2001; Durif et al., 2002: Volkman et al., 1998).

DBS of the subthalamic nucleus (STN) has also been found to have a powerful effect on dyskinesia in individuals with PD (DBSPDSG, 2001; Krack et al., 2003; Ostergaard et al., 2002). A long-term effect has also been reported by Krack and colleagues (2003) at 5-year follow-up. Toda and colleagues (2004) suggest the mechanisms of the effect of STN DBS on reductions in dyskinesia are thought to be a combination of post-operative "reduction in medication and . . . a direct anti-dyskinetic effect" (p. 9).

DBS is also being explored in other forms of dyskinesia. Kosel and colleagues (2007) report on one 62-year-old female with TD due to neuroleptic exposure who underwent bilateral GPi DBS. At 18 months, both dyskinesia and depression were improved.

Bilateral STN DBS has also been described as a treatment for TD, though the effect is difficult to determine from the literature (Sun, Chen, Zhan, Le, & Krahl, 2007).

SWALLOWING IN DYSKINESIA

Epidemiology

The contribution of dyskinesia to swallowing dysfunction in PD is difficult to establish because the dyskinesia is but one of the possible abnormalities in this condition. The relationship of TD to dysphagia is easier to establish, though data are limited. Feve and colleagues (1995) completed clinical examinations of swallowing in 12 patients with TD, although the exact method was not described. Five of 12 (42%) had difficulty swallowing. The condition was described as moderate in four and severe in one based on the presence of aspiration. They speculate that abnormal lowering of the larynx during swallowing could be at least partially responsible for the dysphagia. Another contributor could be the breakdown in swallowing and breathing coordination. That breakdown could result from abnormal oral movements that hinder bolus formation and movement, thereby disrupting the timing of all swallowing events, or from laryngeal dyskinesia that periodically compromises airway protection, or from respiratory dyskinesia that disrupts respiratory timing, or from some combination.

Hayashi and colleagues (1997) report that up to 75% of patients on neuroleptic medications may develop what they call extrapyramidal symptoms, including, but not limited to, dysphagia. This is perhaps the best summary of limited data that suggest dysphagia should be suspected in TD and any other condition that includes dyskinesia among its signs, especially as the condition becomes more severe. In addition, Gregory and colleagues (1992) identified severe dysphagia characterized by aspiration requiring tube feeding when myotomy and epiglottic placation were unsuccessful. This report serves as a reminder that dysphagia can be severe in some cases.

Symptoms

Perhaps the most complete description of swallowing symptoms was provided by patient K. J. described by Bosma in 1986:

1. This individual described the special timing of introducing food into the mouth: "Now I have to race food, carefully selected and arranged on fork or spoon, past my tongue" (p. 21).
2. Food is pushed from the mouth.
3. Food bunches up in the mouth.
4. Drooling is present.
5. Coughing and choking are a problem.
6. Patient is unable to use a straw or suck on a lozenge.

Signs

Most signs appear not to be unique to this condition, so the clinician should be prepared to identify the traditional bolus flow abnormalities. Nonetheless, certain features can be highlighted:

1. Tongue protrusion that pushes food out of the mouth during chewing or efforts to swallow
2. Tongue protrusion and other abnormal lingual movements that otherwise hinder the efficient preparation and posterior movement of the bolus
3. Tongue and jaw movements that hinder getting food into the mouth and efficiently preparing it for swallowing once in the mouth
4. Disrupted coordination of breathing and swallowing with potential for penetration and aspiration; some aspiration events may be silent (Gregory, Smith, & Rudge, 1992)
5. Incoordination of oral and pharyngeal stages of swallow with stasis in valleculae and pyriform sinuses
6. Variability in all signs is likely, presumably because of variability in coordination across swallows

Functional/Quality of Life Consequences

Patients have been forced onto tube feedings and reduced to taking thickened liquids and pureed foods. In general, both are threats to quality of life. The "messy eating" with food falling from the mouth and the unpredictable choking can make eating a socially unsatisfying experience and one to be avoided. The unpredictability can have an especially negative impact on peace of mind. K. J. (Bosma, 1986) described a number of functional and quality of life consequences including:

1. The inability to "savor" food
2. The embarrassment of being offered a lozenge by a helpful stranger and having to try to swallow it without spitting it back up
3. Having to wear clothes that do not show stains
4. Being forced to eat alone
5. Being nervous around new people

Perhaps most tellingly, K. J. said, "I think one of the hardest things about dyskinesia is that no one knows what it is, and as a result, its manifestations generate unlovely attitudes" (p. 22).

Health Consequences

The most dramatic health consequence can be death, and this is probably most likely only in the mentally ill who have been on medication for long periods and have developed severe TD, decreased mental status, and behavioral changes. This may be more likely in patients who require institutionalization. Generally, however, it appears that the swallowing problems, if identified early and if medical treatment is successful, are more inconvenient than life threatening.

Swallowing Evaluation

Chart Review and History

The guidelines in Chapter 4 can be followed. Of special concern in dyskinesia are the following:

1. The medical diagnosis and whether the dyskinesia is TD or part of another condition such as PD.
2. Medications a person has been on, whether it is TD or dyskinesia as part of PD or some other neurologic condition. The phenothiazines are most frequently the cause of TD, but other medications, such as risperidone, have been implicated (Friedman, 1998). And, of course, long-term use of PD medications can cause periods of dyskinesia.
3. Determining whether dyskinesia exists alone or in combination with other abnormalities such as dystonia, rigidity, tremor (frequent), or chorea (less frequent).
4. The pattern or consistency of the dyskinesia during the day. In PD, it may wax and wane, but generally not in TD, although it is possible that the dyskinesia resolves in a small number of cases even without treatment.
5. The length of time each medication has been prescribed.
6. Swallowing consequences and what, if anything, the person has done to control or compensate for them.
7. Medication changes that have been made and their effects on swallowing, if any.
8. Determining what medical treatments are planned or ongoing.
9. Determining if a surgical treatment is planned. This is more likely in those with PD.
10. The relationship of medications and treatments to the swallowing problem.

11. Any pattern the patient recognizes in the severity of the dysphagia and what each patient has tried to help control the problem and with what success. This information may guide the clinician toward what to do and what not to do.

12. Determining if serious choking episodes requiring the Heimlich or other emergency procedures have occurred, when, and with what result.

Clinical Swallow Examination (CSE)

The guidelines in Chapter 5 can be followed. Of special interest in dyskinesia is observing, to the degree possible, the distribution of the dyskinesia across all important swallowing structures, including respiration. Doing so may require careful observation over several seconds or even minutes and special testing such as controlled exhalation and vowel prolongation to support hypotheses about the distribution of the dyskinesia. Requiring maximum performance such as alternate motion rates (AMRs) and vowel prolongation may amplify the dyskinesia, making observation easier.

Also observe, to the degree possible, the presence and distribution of other movement abnormalities, such as dystonia, tremor, rigidity, and chorea. Use a variety of both clinician and patient delivered foods and liquids to:

1. Establish the sign of tongue thrust during swallowing

2. Establish potential difficulty getting food and drink to the mouth because of limb movement abnormality

3. Observe potential variability and discover patterns, if they exist

4. Observe the effects of a variety of compensations as outlined in the Behavioral Treatment section that follows

5. Allow extended observation of swallowing and respiration as when a brisk inhalation occurs while a bolus is in the mouth

Videofluoroscopic Swallow Examination (VFSE)

Videofluoroscopic swallow examination (VFSE) in dyskinesia can be especially valuable by allowing observation of the distribution and effect of dyskinesia. The examination can be completed according to the methodology outlined in Chapter 6. Of special interest in dyskinesia will be:

1. Observation of swallow structure movements with and without swallowing.

2. Observation in support of the strongest possible hypothesis about the interaction of swallowing and respiration. In cases of dyskinesia involving the larynx, lapses in airway protection may result in dysphagia (Feve, Angelard, & St Guily, 1995).

3. Comparison of self-administered and clinician-administered boluses.

4. Observation of compensations as described below in the Behavioral Treatment section.

Videoendoscopic Swallowing Examination

See Chapter 7 for complete details. This exam, perhaps in modified form, may also be of special value in this population. Feve and colleagues (1995) are among those to have identified laryngeal TD, in which dyskinesia causes adduction of the vocal folds with disruptions of breathing. While this phenomenon cannot be observed during swallowing, it can be noted during simple observation and performance of tasks such as vowel prolongation.

Behavioral Treatment

Compensatory Approaches

All the compensations we traditionally have used are included in Chapter 13. They can be reviewed for fit with the individual patient. Variability is a challenge in most movement disorders and no more so than in dyskinesia, so promising any resolution of dysphagia is unrealistic. Nonetheless, compensations are worth trying. To be considered especially are:

1. Head and jaw stabilization, especially in those with a tongue thrust pattern
2. Foods that require minimal chewing
3. Identifying periods when dyskinesia may be less severe, which usually might mean nothing more elaborate than trying to eat without stress or hurry
4. Considering multiple small meals if fatigue heightens the dyskinesia
5. Starting with liquid to moisten the swallowing tube and perhaps reduce the struggle with dry, chunky foods

Rehabilitation Techniques

No evidence for the effect of behavioral treatments is known to us. However, if a patient is facing the unpalatable choices of unappetizing food and liquid preparations or even tube feedings, then we would be tempted to try other techniques under very close supervision, including RMST (p. 83) if there is any hint that a stronger respiratory system would be of potential benefit. LSVT (p. 81) could also be attempted, although, depending on the swallowing signs, the rationale is unclear. Variations of the hard swallow (p. 104), which might help the patient focus on careful, effortful swallowing, are another possibility. If increased dysphagia is observed, then this method is obviously to be discontinued.

SUMMARY

Dysphagia due to dyskinesia is a challenging condition for the dysphagia clinician because compensations rather than rehabilitation appear to be most appropriate. Nonetheless, a role is clear in identifying the swallowing abnormalities and their possible causes and advising about the safest, most adequate, and pleasurable nutrition and hydration possible. In those cases where dyskinesia appears as part of another primary movement disorder (e.g., PD, dystonia), the rehabilitation approaches outlined in Chapter 14 may be of use. Additionally, Chapter 15 on PD and Chapter 18 on dystonia may be useful in some cases.

22 Tremor

Definition

Tremor in its purest form is *rhythmic oscillation* and ranks among the most frequent movement disorders. Fernandez and colleagues (2007) describe tremor as "involuntary, regular, rhythmic, oscillatory, to-and-from movements" (p. 47). Tremor occurs in persons without neurologic disease and is called *physiologic tremor*. Abnormal tremor comes in a variety of forms, with each of the forms having a slightly different but overlapping frequency. Tremors can be *resting,* *postural*, or *action* (or kinetic). They most frequently involve the limbs or structures of head and neck but can involve the entire body or any part, including the swallowing structures. Resting tremor is a cardinal sign of Parkinson's disease (PD) as discussed in Chapter 15. Action tremor is a principal feature of cerebellar disease (Chapter 19) and can occur in multiple sclerosis (MS) and a variety of other conditions. Postural tremor is less diagnostic and may be seen in PD and other conditions. Tremor may be associated with a variety of conditions and etiologies, as suggested by Manyam (2004), who discusses 18 additional classes of tremor as seen in Table 22-1.

Table 22–1. Eighteen additional classes of tremor discussed by Manyam (2004)

Type	Description
Physiological	Found in normal persons, seldom symptomatic except on finely skilled tasks
Cortical tremor	Rare tremor usually resulting from generalized brain damage; described as having the characteristics of cortical myoclonus
Cerebellar tremor	Often begins in progressive neurologic disease involving the cerebellum as terminal tremor, which is manifest on finger to nose testing as the finger reaches the target; evolves to occur during purposeful movement; not present at rest
Dystonic tremor	Probably an unsatisfactory label for an irregular tremor that appears in a dystonic body part

continues

Table 22–1. *continued*	
Type	**Description**
Food-induced tremor	Tremor associated with a variety of foods and beverages with alcohol, coffee, and other "stimulating" drinks often implicated
Drug-induced tremor	Some drugs such as antidepressants, cardiac medications, dopamine receptor-blocking medications, and immunosuppressants can cause tremor; one form, so-called rabbit syndrome, involves tremor primarily of the lips
Toxin-induced tremor	Exposure to a variety of heavy metals, insecticides, and solvents may cause tremor
Holmes tremor	This is a slow tremor, rate below 4.5 oscillations per second, occurring at rest and during action; also called midbrain tremor because of the frequent involvement of the midbrain when this tremor is present
Primary orthostatic tremor	Also called shaky leg syndrome, this tremor is present in the legs upon standing
Palatal tremor	Formerly called palatal myoclonus, this is a slow tremor of approximately two per second; divided into symptomatic and essential forms with symptomatic tremor often involving other bulbar structures in addition to the palate
Peripheral neuropathy-associated tremor	Peripheral neuropathy, as may occur with diabetes, alcoholism, and kidney disease, can cause tremor
Psychogenic tremors	Can occur in a variety of psychogenic disorders and is characterized by acute onset, irregularity, and frequent remissions
Rest tremor	An odd addition to the list of tremors, rest tremor occurs when a body part is at rest and supported
Stroke-associated tremor	Tremor following thalamic stroke is one of best known; may occur immediately or after a delay
Tremor in systemic diseases	Tremor can be included among the signs of AIDS, Wilson's disease (see Chapter 23), hypoxia (as in Lance-Adams syndrome), and a variety of other diseases such as thyroid disease
Task-specific tremor	Tremor occurring during the performance of skilled tasks such as handwriting; probably a variant of essential tremor
Posttraumatic tremor	Tremor can result from traumatic injury to cerebellum, thalamus, midbrain, basal ganglia, and other structures
Vocal tremor	For some reason, tremor of the vocal folds has earned its own spot in the list; vocal tremor most easily detected on prolongation of a vowel, usually in combination with tremor in other systems; probably a variant of essential tremor

Note. From "Uncommon Forms of Tremor," by B. V. Manyam, 2004, in R. L. Watts and W. C. Koller (Eds.), *Movement Disorders: Neurologic Principles and Practice* (2nd ed., pp. 459–480), New York: McGraw-Hill. Reprinted with permission.

Tremor is typically absent during sleep. Different tremor types occurring in isolation or as part of a larger symptom complex, as in PD and MS, may respond to medications. Deep brain stimulation (DBS) is now employed in many severe cases of tremor. Tremor, especially if induced by action, can significantly alter function, including swallowing if the structures of the swallowing mechanism are involved. Tremor is generally very difficult to treat. Tremor may be associated with a variety of clinical conditions including PD, *essential tremor* (ET), cerebellar disorders, *Holmes' tremor*, *dystonic tremor*, *enhanced physiologic tremor*, *orthostatic tremor*, and *neuropathic tremor* (Fernandez, Rodriguez, Skidmore, & Okun, 2007).

The most frequent tremor type is so-called ET. ET, also known as *familial tremor*, has a frequency of 4–8 Hz (although higher rates may be encountered) and can be worsened by fatigue or strong emotion. The tremor is unaccompanied by other signs of neurologic deficit and indeed, if other signs are present, ET is an unlikely diagnosis. The exception, of course, is that person who has two neurologic diagnoses in which tremor is a sign.

Signs/Diagnostic Criteria

Tremor may be *resting* (present when a body part is supported and at rest), *postural* (present when a body part is held against gravity), *action* (present during performance of an activity), and/or *intentional* (a variation of action in which tremor worsens as a target is approached).

Tremor rates across these types overlap. The usual range of rates is 1 to 18 Hz. In some conditions such as cerebellar tremor, frequencies may vary by body part, being higher in the hands and arms than in the trunk. A tremor at 4–8 Hz, most prominent when the person tries to maintain a posture, is the cardinal feature in ET. Tremor at rest and during action can also occur, however, not only in ET but in other tremors as well.

All types of tremor are more likely in hands and fingers, and, according to Fernandez and colleagues (2007), the next most likely sites are the tongue, head, jaw, legs, and trunk. In ET, the initial tremor is most usually in the hands bilaterally, although unilateral onset is typical. ET may occasionally begin in the head, tongue, or larynx, and it may appear in the bulbar structures prior to appearing in the hands.

Tremor can respond to a variety of manipulations. Alcohol and bracing, as when one rests his head on a hand, can alter ET. Discontinuing the cause of tremor (such as medications) can sometimes reduce tremor. Some but not all tremors disappear during sleep.

Mild frontal cognitive deficits may accompany ET, and a variety of other neurologic signs may accompany most other forms of tremor, especially those in which tremor is only part of a neurologic syndrome such as PD.

It is beyond this book's scope to list all diagnostic criteria for the various forms of tremor. In most cases, they can be inferred. Criteria in ET, the most frequent of the tremor types, include "postural tremor . . . that worsens with action" and the absence of other neurologic disease such as PD, anxiety, alcoholism, or other causes of tremor (Cersosimo & Koller, 2004, p. 437). A secondary criterion is postural tremor of hands and head in the absence of other, alternative explanations for tremor, such as hyperthyroidism.

Evolution

ET can appear at any time in childhood or adulthood but is usually seen in the late 20s and the later 30s and beyond. Some cases of childhood onset have been reported. Progress is usually relentless and spreads from the structures where it initially appeared to others. For example, it may expand from the arms and hands to include the head and then the lips, tongue, palate, pharynx, and larynx. The tremor may increase in amplitude as well. With time, the tremor becomes more and more obvious and has greater functional impact.

Tremor may worsen over time in a variety of other conditions, including toxin- and drug-induced tremors, as well as in systemic disease. Onset may be relatively immediate in stroke and trauma but may also be delayed, sometimes for years.

Epidemiology

ET is often inherited, but other factors may play a role in many cases. Prevalence is estimated at approximately 1074 per 100,000 persons in the fourth decade and later according to Cersosimo and Koller, (2004), who also note that 5 million adults in the United States over 40 may have the disorder. Men may be slightly more likely than women to have ET. Tremor is also frequent in PD unless one has the rigid-akinetic form of the disease. Similarly, tremor is frequent in cerebellar disease. Other forms of tremor are less common.

Evaluation

Medical Assessment

A variety of scales for quantifying the distribution of tremor have been developed.

Cersosimo and Koller (2004) include three scales, two for the practitioner and one for self-report, in their discussion of ET. All scales are five-point, equal-appearing, interval scales with 0 being assigned in the absence of tremor and 4 being assigned to severe, disabling tremor. The two scales for clinicians are used to evaluate tremor generally and while pouring water with one and then the other hand. The self-assessment scales have the patient score tremor during a variety of activities (see Table 22–2) using a five-point scale.

Table 22–2. Activities scored for self-assessment of severity of tremor

Tremor
Speaking/phonation
Feeding (other than liquids)
Drinking
Hygiene
Dressing
Writing
Working
Fine movements
Embarrassment
Handwriting with strategy (patient chooses)
Handwriting without strategy
Drawing
Spiral
Connecting two straight lines with a straight line

Note. Swallowing is not scored. Establishing the effect of tremor and swallowing falls to the swallowing clinician. From "Essential Tremor," by M. G. Cersosimo and W. C. Koller, 2004, in: R. L. Watts and W. C. Koller (Eds.), *Movement Disorders: Neurologic Principles and Practice* (2nd ed., pp. 431–458), New York: McGraw-Hill. Reprinted with permission.

The greatest evaluation challenge in tremor is to identify which of the multiple types it is. A good history is the first step. Family history, medical history, history of medication use, and exposure to toxins are all likely to be informative. Determining the type and distribution of tremor, whether resting, postural or static and whether in extremities, bulbar musculature, or trunk are also first steps. Identifying the coexisting abnormalities such as rigidity, spasticity, dystonia, dementia, behavioral abnormality, and psychiatric is also important.

The dysphagia clinician charged with evaluating the swallow effects of tremor would do well to become familiar with the multiple medications, systemic diseases, and other influences on tremor. Doing so makes the clinician a more effective health care team member by allowing her to recognize that tremor arises from multiple causes and the cause can influence treatment and expectations.

Medical Treatment

In general, tremor is resistant to treatment. There are exceptions, of course. Zesiewicz and colleagues (2005) have written a useful survey of the medical/surgical treatments of ET. Medications such as propranolol and primidone may have some therapeutic effect in ET, although an effect is less likely on vocal tremor.

Alcohol often has a dramatic therapeutic effect on ET, especially early on, but does nothing to stem the condition and may actually make it more severe. Patients often have discovered alcohol as a self-medication. Medications, in general, have not been of demonstrated efficacy in most other forms of tremor.

Withdrawing or reducing the dosages of medications causing tremor can be helpful. Medical management of psychogenic tremor can be useful. Behavioral, rehabilitative methods of tremor treatment are usually ineffective.

Surgical Treatment

DBS of the thalamus, most commonly of the ventral intermedius nucleus (VIM), may suppress some forms of tremor, especially in the limbs contralateral to the surgery. Generally, DBS is considered only after medical treatments have failed.

Marrosu and colleagues (2007) report improvement in cerebellar postural tremor and in dysphagia in three patients with MS following vagal nerve stimulation. Botulinum toxin injections have also been used with a variety of tremors, including dystonic tremor. Gamma knife thalamotomy is still offered in some centers (Kondziolka et al., 2008).

Effects on Swallowing

Botulinum toxin injections to improve vocal tremor, especially of suprahyoid musculature, may cause dysphagia (Merati et al., 2005). Botulinum toxin injections to the thyroarytenoid musculature seem to be less frequently associated with dysphagia (Merati et al., 2005), though dysphagia has been reported in 3 of 13 patients (23%) at 2 weeks post-injection; however, it had improved in two by 6 weeks (Adler et al, 2004).

Kondziolka and colleagues (2008) report only one mild postsurgery case of dysphagia in 31 patients whose medically intractable ET was treated with gamma knife thalamotomy. Alusi et al. (2001) report 2 of 24 MS patients (8%) were dysphagic after stereotactic lesional surgery, with resolution in one of these cases.

SWALLOWING IN TREMOR

Epidemiology

Dysphagia would seem to be relatively infrequent in tremor involving the head and swallowing structures unless the tremor is severe, generalized to all the bulbar structures, or part of a more complex set of neurologic deficits such as dystonia, spasticity, or rigidity. Nonetheless, it can occur, and its locus in the oral or pharyngeal stages or resulting from airway protection failure is dependent on the distribution of the tremor. For example, vocal tremor appears more likely to be associated with dysphagia than lingual tremor. Lingual tremor appears more likely to induce dysphagia than facial tremor. (Zesiewicz et al., 2005). Merati and colleagues (2005) remind us that vocal or laryngeal tremor is actually an inappropriate term, as laryngeal tremor is likely to be accompanied by tremor in the extrinsic laryngeal musculature, pharynx, tongue, and respiratory mechanism. One might speculate therefore that at least mild dysphagia is likely in tremor of the bulbar structures, especially with increasing severity in distribution and amplitude. Of course, upper extremity tremor is likely to complicate moving food and drink to the mouth, which can create coordination problems in the oral stage, which in turn may disrupt pharyngeal, laryngeal, and respiratory coordination.

Symptoms

Because dysphagia is relatively infrequent in tremor unless severe, widely distributed, or accompanied by other neuro-logic abnormalities, prospective studies are scarce, and indeed we could discover none. In general, the clinician can expect that any of the signs reported for any of the other movement abnormalities may be reported by patients with tremor. Drawing from our own clinical experiences, we can report the following swallowing symptoms:

1. Difficulty keeping bolus in the mouth
2. Drooling
3. Food sticking in the mouth or throat
4. Coughing and choking

Signs

Similarly, signs are underreported in the literature. Any of the signs reported in careful studies of other movement disorders can occur in tremor. Again, based our clinical experiences, we can highlight the following signs.

Oral Stage

Signs include:

1. Poor containment of the bolus, especially in rabbit syndrome or other serious tremor of lips and jaw
2. Haphazard formation of the bolus in the oral cavity
3. Inefficient, hesitant movement of the bolus posteriorly to initiate the pharyngeal stage of swallowing

Pharyngeal Stage

Pharyngeal stage signs may include:

1. Inefficient and incomplete movement of the bolus through the pharynx
2. Residue in the valleculae and pyriforms

3. Variable signs from swallow to swallow, depending probably on timing of tremor with bolus movement
4. Discoordination of the swallow and respiration; recall that tremor of the respiratory structures may be more common than reported

Laryngeal Stage

These signs may include the following:

1. Penetration that is variable in its depth and whether or not it is forced out of the larynx during or after the swallow
2. Less frequent aspiration and variability in its severity when it does occur
3. Retained sense of when material has entered the airway, so infrequent silent aspiration

Functional/Quality of Life Consequences

Again, the full range of such consequences can be expected. Tremor, however, whether or not it is accompanied by dysphagia, is often embarrassing and therefore persons with tremor may avoid eating in public and even with family. The variability of their swallowing competence can leave them insecure because they cannot predict what foods, liquids, or conditions are more likely to be associated with difficulty swallowing.

Health Consequences

Pulmonary consequences, malnutrition, dehydration, and other consequences reported in the other movement disorder chapters are less likely in the tremor population. Swallowing made worse by a surgical treatment for the tremor may be more likely to result in serious adverse health consequences.

Swallow Evaluation

Chart Review and History

The history and chart review requirements are described in Chapter 4. Of special interest to the diagnosis of tremor is to determine its distribution across the structures important to swallowing and to determine if the tremor is ET or part of a more generalized neurologic syndrome. It is especially important to seek the following information:

1. Date of onset of tremor
2. Location at onset, whether one or both limbs, head, or other structures with special attention to lips, tongue, larynx, and respiratory mechanism
3. Course of tremor, which means involvement of other structures and any changes in frequency and amplitude of tremor in the first one affected and all other structures
4. Presence of any other neurologic abnormality such as changes in tone, strength, or coordination
5. Influences such as fatigue, emotion, and alcohol on tremor
6. Medical treatments underway or planned, and if completed, effect on swallowing and eating generally
7. Family history of tremor and other neurologic disease
8. Impact of tremor on quality of life including functional status
9. Influence on getting food and drink to mouth
10. Influence on chewing and swallowing

11. Any "tricks," such as resting head in hands, that help with eating and swallowing
12. Presence of drooling
13. Choking, coughing, food sticking
14. Any other consequences of swallowing abnormality

Clinical Swallow Examination (CSE)

The clinical swallow examination (CSE) may be especially important in tremor, especially ET, because the functional impact of the condition may not be readily appreciated from VFSE or videoendoscopic examination. The general procedures are described in Chapter 5. Two goals should be achieved. One is establishing the distribution of tremor, especially in the structures of the head, neck, and respiratory mechanism:

1. Head tremor can be observed.
2. Lip tremor can be observed.
3. Jaw tremor can be observed.
4. Tongue tremor can be accentuated by having the patient hold tongue protrusion.
5. Velopharyngeal tremor can be observed with a light while patient is instructed merely to remain silent.
6. Laryngeal tremor can be inferred from prolonged vowel prolongation and may possibly be palpated in some cases.
7. Respiratory tremor is hard to see but may be inferred from feeling the respiratory muscles and from patient performance on nonvoiced exhalation so that the larynx is not approximated. Of course, if tremulous, the folds may move, thereby affecting the airstream, so this test is far from perfect. It is, however, an alternative

to expensive and frequently unavailable instrumental testing. Again, in some cases respiratory tremor may be palpated and/or visualized.

8. A rough approximation of tremor frequency can be made perceptually. Such calculations, of course, are prone to error, both of measurement and of interpretation, but are worth pursuing nonetheless.
9. Because tremor often coexists with other movement abnormalities, especially in tremor disorders where tremor is but one part of the syndrome, inferences about abnormal tone, strength, and coordination using whatever tools one normally uses for such inferences are also essential.

A second goal is observing usual and compensated eating and drinking:

1. Watching eating and drinking using whatever method the patient typically uses (e.g., finger foods, weighted silverware, arm weights, use of a straw) is also important.
2. Having the patient with head and other head and neck tremor repeat liquid and solid swallows with the head and jaw braced may also yield treatment dividends, although the usual patient has tried all the common sense compensations.

Videofluoroscopic Swallow Examination (VFSE)

We prefer the videofluoroscopic swallow examination (VFSE) for tremor patients because it allows for clear observation of tremor in all swallowing structures, though the larynx can be a challenge to view. The anterior-posterior (AP) view may be helpful in this regard. In our experience, it is remarkable how infrequently tremor of any type influences the swallow. More commonly, we have encountered difficulty getting food and drink to the mouth. Once inside the mouth, the usual patient does normally or reasonably well. There are exceptions, of course, and we have seen them. Therefore, the traditional examination described in Chapter 6, with special attention to using a few seconds in the beginning to simply record and then observe the distribution of the tremor, is recommended. Of additional, special interest may be the following:

1. Contrast swallowing with patient bracing head and chin and without such bracing
2. Contrasting more and less solid food items
3. Contrasting straw and cup swallowing, if possible
4. Bolus size variation can also be informative
5. Contrasting clinician and patient provided boluses

In our experience, if a patient has difficulty, she most commonly begins doing things such as excessively moving the bolus in the mouth until she feels she can safely swallow. This maneuver may slow the swallow but generally improve overall swallow biomechanics. However, in some cases, a maladaptive struggle creeps into the oral stage with negative impact on the pharyngeal stage and on penetration and aspiration.

In general, the examination is a search for the best compensations, because no behavioral method is of proven effect. Furthermore, it is difficult to even

hypothesize about sensible rehabilitation approaches.

Videoendoscopic Swallow Examination

Complete details for the videoendoscopic swallow examination are found in Chapter 7. Videoendoscopy may be of particular diagnostic value when direct visualization of the larynx in needed, such as in cases of possible pharyngeal, laryngeal, and velopharyngeal tremor.

Behavioral Treatment

Compensatory Approaches

In cases of tremor uncomplicated by other abnormalities of tone, strength, or coordination, compensatory methods will be the treatments of choice (see Chapter 13). Even these are likely to be of greatest benefit if medical or surgical treatments have been successful in reducing tremor. In the case of such a treatment's abolishing tremor, any behavioral approach will be unnecessary of course, though tremor in the bulbar structures is often uninfluenced by surgical approaches and may even become more severely involved. The following compensations may be of special interest:

1. Weights on the ankles and wrists may reduce tremor amplitude and improve getting food and drink to the mouth.
2. Weighted utensils may help in a similar fashion.
3. Postural adjustments such as stabilizing the head may be useful. A useful experiment is to have the patient eat

while resting her head against a high-back chair.

4. Resting the head in the hand, depending on distribution of the tremor, may help chewing and swallowing.

5. Food consistency and liquid viscosity may also be changed with a therapeutic effect.

6. Occasionally, merely reassuring a patient that the swallow is safe (if it is, of course) can have a therapeutic effect.

Rehabilitation Techniques

No rehabilitative technique is of demonstrated efficacy for dysphagia secondary to tremor. If weakness is also present, then any of the strengthening methods outlined in Chapter 14 can be tried. We wish it were otherwise, but our experience is that tremor is often worsened by some of the treatments that require increased effort, such as the hard swallow.

SUMMARY

Tremor is a complex condition to discuss. As a sign, tremor may exist in relative isolation (e.g., ET) or with a variety of other neurological signs in a diverse number of conditions (e.g., PD, MS). Dysphagia may occur in patients with tremor, particularly if it is severe, the distribution involves structures of the swallowing mechanism, or it is part of a more pervasive neurologic disease.

23 Wilson's Disease

WILSON'S DISEASE

Definition

Wilson's disease (WD) is a rare autosomal-recessive genetic disease associated with copper accumulation in the liver, brain, and eyes due to an impairment of gastrointestinal elimination of this material. Genetically, the abnormal gene appears to be located on chromosome 13. Signs of liver disease may precede or follow nervous system signs. Regardless of order, eye and nervous system signs often appear at about the same time. Machado and colleagues (2006) identify what they call "three primary syndromes," depending on whether dystonia, ataxia, or parkinsonian signs predominate (p. 2194). Machado et al. also identify two other forms of the disease, depending on age at onset: the Westphal-Strümpell form as occurring later, often when the person is 20 or older, and a juvenile form that occurs earlier.

Signs/Diagnostic Criteria

Psychiatric, neurologic, and hepatic signs occur in various combinations and in varying orders. The *Kayser-Fleisher ring* resulting from copper deposits in the eye is pathognomonic of the condition (Pfeif-fer, 2004) and commonly occurs in combination with neurologic signs, but is not inevitable. Machado and colleagues (2006) tabulated the neurologic signs in 119 patients with WD, as shown in Table 23-1. Dysarthria occurs frequently in WD and has been reported in over 90% of unselected patients with neurologic signs in some studies (Machado et al., 2006; Oder et al., 1991; Wang et al., 2005). Dysphagia appears to occur less frequently than dysarthria, though this has received little attention. Other frequent, early neurologic signs may include gait abnormalities, dystonia, *riscus sardonicus* (smile-like grimace), bradykinesia, tremor, and chorea. Micrographia, masked facies, and drooling may also be present (Machado et al., 2006). Dystonia may be most likely in those with early onset of the disease (i.e., age 10 or earlier).

In some individuals, behavioral and/or psychiatric decline may also be early signs, including depression, lability, and irritability. More serious abnormalities such as catatonia and mania may also occur, and hospitalization for psychiatric problems has been reported. Cognitive impairment may also occur.

Kayser-Fleischer rings, evidence of liver disease, a family history of similar signs, and laboratory values, including abnormal copper in the urine and low serum copper, support the diagnosis.

Table 23–1. Neurologic signs and their frequency in 119 patients with Wilson's disease (WD)

Neurological Manifestations	Total Number of Patients	Percent of Patients
Dysarthria	109	91
Gait abnormalities	89	75
Dystonia	82	69
Riscus sardonicus	86	72
Bradykinesia	68	58
Rigidity	78	66
Postural instability	54	49
Resting tremor	6	5
Postural tremor	65	55
Cerebellar disturbance (other than dysarthria and tremor)	33	28
Dysphagia	59	50
Chorea	19	16
Athetosis	17	14

Note. From "Neurological Manifestations in Wilson's Disease. Report of 119 Cases," by A. Machado, H. F. Chien, M. Deguti, E. Cancado, R. S. Azevedo, et al., 2006, *Movement Disorders, 21*(12), pp. 2192–2196. Copyright 1996. Reprinted with the permission of Wiley-Liss, Inc., a subsidiary of John Wiley & Sons, Inc.

Evolution

Signs worsen with time. Ropper and Brown (2005) observe that "[t]he patient becomes mute, immobile, extremely rigid, dystonic, and slowed mentally, the latter usually being a late and variable effect" (p. 831). Dysphagia generally worsens with time and may contribute to patient death.

Epidemiology

Occurrence of the disease is estimated to be 1 per 30,000 but increases in areas where consanguinity is present. In a sample of 119 patients, average age at onset was 19.6 years, with a range of 7 to 37 years, although onset in the fifth decade has been reported. One in four siblings of a patient with Wilson's disease will inherit the condition. It is more common in women than in men (Machado et al., 2006).

Medical/Surgical Treatment

Reducing dietary copper; chelation with medication, primarily D-penicillamine; and, in some cases, liver transplantation (Wang et al., 2005) are the treatments of choice. Wang and colleagues (2005) report improved neurologic status including swallowing function following liver transplantation.

SWALLOWING IN WD

Epidemiology

Bulbar signs, including dysphagia, can occur early in Wilson's disease, and if left untreated, may well further compromise patient health. Machado and colleagues (2006) reported dysphagia in 50% of 119 patients and dysarthria in more than 90%. This may well be an underestimation in the case of dysphagia, as most patients do not seem to have had instrumental examination, and instead the presence of signs were determined at history or clinical exam. It is probably safe to assume that patients with WD and neurologic signs will likely have dysphagia sometime during the disease's course.

Symptoms

We discovered no systematic study of swallowing symptoms in WD. Gulyas and Salazar-Grueso (1988) described a single patient with complaint of difficulty swallowing for 20 years and described coughing during meals and food sticking in her throat that cleared with water. In our experience, patients often deny symptoms. Given the behavioral, psychiatric, and cognitive disturbances that frequently are part of this disorder, the clinician would do well to confirm patient report with that of a caregiver or other member of the medical team and to complete a clinical swallow examination (CSE)if there is any suspicion of dysphagia, particularly in the setting of other bulbar dysfunction.

Signs

A small literature describing the swallowing signs in WD has emerged. Wilson's first patient had dysphagia otherwise undescribed (Wilkins & Brody, 1971). Da Silva-Junior and colleagues (2007) suggest that the signs in WD with prominent parkinsonian signs generally can be expected to have signs similar to those in PD and report the following signs based on scintigraphy:

1. Slowed oral transit of the bolus
2. Greater than normal oral residuals
3. Pharyngeal transit within normal limits
4. Pharyngeal residual within normal limits

Gulyas and Salazar-Grueso (1988) reported VFSE results on one patient. Her signs were:

1. Normal oral stage
2. Vallecular residue
3. Pyriform sinus residue

4. Aspiration from the valleculae after the swallow was complete
5. Clearing of material with repeat swallows

Functional/Quality of Life Consequences

To our knowledge, functional status and quality of life have not been systematically studied in WD. Patients unaware of the dysphagia may suffer no consequences, although their caregivers doubtless do.

Health Consequences

Fatal choking, pulmonary illness, weight loss, dehydration, and malnutrition are all possible health consequences.

Evaluation

History and Chart Review

Chapter 4 contains a complete description of the history and chart review procedures. Of special concern in WD are the following:

1. Evidence of any eating and swallowing problems
2. Evidence of health consequences of swallowing problems
3. Evidence of functional and quality of life consequences of swallowing problems
4. Evidence of behavioral abnormalities
5. Evidence of psychiatric abnormalities
6. Evidence of cognitive abnormalities
7. Relevant data on whether motor problems are ataxic, Parkinsonian, and/or dystonic

8. Planned or completed medical and surgical treatments
9. Effects of those treatments on swallowing
10. Evidence of patient compliance with recommendations by other health care providers

Clinical Swallow Examination (CSE)

The CSE is completely described in Chapter 5, and that chapter can guide the examination of persons with WD. Of special consideration is the following:

1. Effect of any behavioral abnormalities on swallowing
2. Effect of any psychiatric abnormalities on swallowing
3. Effect of any cognitive abnormalities on swallowing
4. Evidence on exam of the relative predominance of ataxic, parkinsonian, or dystonic abnormalities on swallowing
5. Indications that patient recognizes any deficits
6. Evidence that patient is interested in eating and other activities

Videofluoroscopic Swallow Examination (VFSE)

The videofluoroscopic swallow examination (VFSE) is described in Chapter 6. Of special concern for the individual with WD will be collecting data, which will allow at least a hypothesis about whether the pattern of swallowing abnormality is predominately ataxic, parkinsonian, dystonic, or some mixture. This is most simply done by comparing the patient's signs with those described in these three conditions in earlier chapters. In our experience, the patient with WD can be very complex, so these determinations are not easily made. However, attempting to do so may guide treatment decisions.

Attending to whether oropharyngeal activities are coordinated with laryngeal and respiratory activities is also important. In the absence of special instrumentation, this relationship may be difficult to discern, but insightful clinicians can often create reasonably accurate hypotheses once prompted to look for evidence of coordination.

Be sure to examine the full range of compensations (see Chapter 13). Attempt to guarantee that pre- and posttreatment examinations are completed whenever possible.

Videoendoscopic Swallow Examination

The videoendoscopic swallow examination is described in Chapter 7.

Treatment

Successful medical or surgical treatment may obviate the need for swallowing treatment. In the absence of such success, compensations and even rehabilitation may be appropriate, despite the absence of data on effect.

Compensatory Approaches

The entire range of compensatory approaches described in Chapter 13 may be applicable; thus, they will not be repeated here. The reader is directed to that chapter, as well as Chapters 10 (Principles of Compensatory Treatments) and Chapter 12 (General Treatment Considerations) for more details. Of special consideration in WD will be compliance, given the high

likelihood of behavioral, psychiatric, and cognitive abnormalities. In general, the recommendation of compensations will need to be acted upon or at least monitored by family/caregivers, especially as the disease progresses and swallowing difficulties become more severe.

Rehabilitation Techniques

The selection of rehabilitation techniques may vary depending on whether signs are more related to ataxia, parkinsonism, or dystonia. It may well be that the entire range of techniques listed in Chapter 14 will be appropriate. However, strengthening treatments may be the least appropriate for many patients. Also, treatments such as the supraglottic swallow may simply be too complex for many patients to master. Additionally, in our experience, the primarily dystonic type of WD is the most difficult to treat behaviorally. Of special use in this condition may be the following:

1. LSVT (p. 81)
2. Hard swallow in its various permutations (p. 104)
3. Mendelsohn maneuver (p. 94)

SUMMARY

WD was assigned a separate chapter because of the tremendous variability that exists in the presentation of patients. That variability makes discussions of evaluation and treatment especially difficult. We have provided special emphasis for assessment and treatments, but it may be that the next person we see will convince us we should have emphasized something different. Regardless, clinicians must be alert to the possibility of dysphagia in patients with WD and neurologic involvement, particularly when other evidence of bulbar dysfunction is present (e.g., dysarthria).

Appendix A

The SWAL-QOL Survey

The SWAL-QOL SURVEY

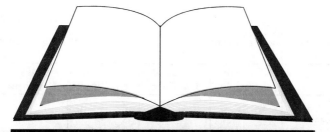

**Understanding
Quality of Life
in Swallowing Disorders**

Instructions for Completing the SWAL-QOL Survey

This questionnaire is designed to find out how your swallowing problem has been affecting your day-to-day quality of life.

Please take the time to carefully read and answer each question. Some questions may look like others, but each one is different.

Here's an <u>example</u> of how the questions in the survey will look.

1. In the last month how often have you experiences each of the symptoms below.

	All of the time	Most of the time	Some of the time	A little of the time	None of the time
Feel weak	1	2	3	4	5

Thank you for your help in taking part in this survey!

IMPORTANT NOTE: We understand that you may have a number of physical problems. Sometimes it is hard to separate these from swallowing difficulties, but we hope that you can do your best to concentrate *only* on your *swallowing problem.* Thank you for your efforts in completing this questionnaire.

1. Below are some general statements that people with *swallowing problems* might mention. In the last month, **how true** have the following statements been for you.

(circle one number on each line)

	Very much true	Quite a bit true	Somewhat true	A little true	Not at all true
Dealing with my swallowing problem is very difficult.	1	2	3	4	5
My swallowing problem is a major distraction in my life.	1	2	3	4	5

2. Below are aspects of day-to-day eating that people with *swallowing problems* sometimes talk about. In the last month, **how true** have the following statements been for you?

(circle one number on each line)

	Very much true	Quite a bit true	Somewhat true	A little true	Not at all true
Most days, I don't care if I eat or not.	1	2	3	4	5
It takes me longer to eat than other people.	1	2	3	4	5
I'm rarely hungry anymore.	1	2	3	4	5
It takes me forever to eat a meal.	1	2	3	4	5
I don't enjoy eating anymore.	1	2	3	4	5

3. Below are some physical problems that people with **swallowing problems** sometimes experience. In the last month, **how often** you have experienced each problem as a result of your swallowing problem?

(circle one number on each line)

	Almost always	Often	Sometimes	Hardly ever	Never
Coughing	1	2	3	4	5
Choking when you eat food	1	2	3	4	5
Choking when you take liquids	1	2	3	4	5
Having thick saliva or phlegm	1	2	3	4	5
Gagging	1	2	3	4	5
Drooling	1	2	3	4	5
Problems chewing	1	2	3	4	5
Having excess saliva or phlegm	1	2	3	4	5
Having to clear your throat	1	2	3	4	5
Food sticking in your throat	1	2	3	4	5
Food sticking in your mouth	1	2	3	4	5
Food or liquid dribbling out of your mouth	1	2	3	4	5
Food or liquid coming out your nose	1	2	3	4	5
Coughing food or liquid out of your mouth when it gets stuck	1	2	3	4	5

4. Next, please answer a few questions about how your **swallowing problem** has affected your diet and eating in the last month.

(circle one number on each line)

	Strongly agree	Agree	Uncertain	Disagree	Strongly disagree
Figuring out what I can and can't eat is a problem for me.	1	2	3	4	5
It is difficult to find foods that I both like and can eat.	1	2	3	4	5

5. In the last month, **how often** have the following statements about communication applied to you because of your *swallowing problem*?

(circle one number on each line)

	All of the time	Most of the time	Some of the time	A little of the time	None of the time
People have a hard time understanding me.	1	2	3	4	5
It's been difficult for me to speak clearly.	1	2	3	4	5

6. Below are some concerns that people with *swallowing problems* sometimes mention. In the last month, **how often** have you experienced each feeling?

(circle one number on each line)

	Almost always	Often	Sometimes	Hardly ever	Never
I fear I may start choking when I eat food.	1	2	3	4	5
I worry about getting pneumonia.	1	2	3	4	5
I am afraid of choking when I drink liquids.	1	2	3	4	5
I never know when I am going to choke.	1	2	3	4	5

7. In the last month, how often have the following statements **been true** for you because of your *swallowing problem*?

(circle one number on each line)

	Always true	Often true	Sometimes true	Hardly ever true	Never true
My swallowing problem depresses me.	1	2	3	4	5
Having to be so careful when I eat or drink annoys me.	1	2	3	4	5
I've been discouraged by my swallowing problem.	1	2	3	4	5
My swallowing problem frustrates me.	1	2	3	4	5
I get impatient dealing with my swallowing problem.	1	2	3	4	5

8. Think about your social life in the last month. How strongly would you agree or disagree with the following statements?

(circle one number on each line)

	Strongly agree	Agree	Uncertain	Disagree	Strongly disagree
I do not go out to eat because of my swallowing problem.	1	2	3	4	5
My swallowing problem makes it hard to have a social life.	1	2	3	4	5
My usual work or leisure activities have changed because of my swallowing problem.	1	2	3	4	5
Social gatherings (like holidays or get-togethers) are not enjoyable because of my swallowing problem.	1	2	3	4	5
My role with family and friends has changed because of my swallowing problem.	1	2	3	4	5

9. In the last month, **how often** have you experienced each of the following physical symptoms?

(circle one number on each line)

	All of the time	Most of the time	Some of the time	A little of the time	None of the time
Feel weak?	1	2	3	4	5
Have trouble falling asleep?	1	2	3	4	5
Feel tired?	1	2	3	4	5
Have trouble staying asleep?	1	2	3	4	5
Feel exhausted?	1	2	3	4	5

10. Do you now take any food or liquid through a feeding tube?

(circle one)

No 1

Yes.. 2

11. Please circle the letter of the one description below that best describes the consistency or texture of the food you have been eating most often in the last week.

Circle one:

A. Circle this one if you are eating a full normal diet, which would include a wide variety of foods, including hard to chew items like steak, carrots, bread, salad, and popcorn.

B. Circle this one if you are eating soft, easy to chew foods like casseroles, canned fruits, soft cooked vegetables, ground meat, or cream soups.

C. Circle this one if you are eating food that is put through a blender or food processor or anything that is like pudding or pureed foods.

D. Circle this one if you take most of your nutrition by tube, but sometimes eat ice cream, pudding, apple sauce, or other pleasure foods.

E. Circle this one if you take all of your nourishment through a tube.

12. **Please circle the letter** of the one description below that best describes the consistency of liquids you have been drinking most often in the last week.

Circle one:

A.   Circle this if you drink liquids such as water, milk, tea, fruit juice, and coffee.

B.   Circle this if the majority of liquids you drink are thick, like tomato juice or apricot nectar. Such thick liquids drip off your spoon in a slow steady stream when you turn it upside down.

C.   Circle this if your liquids are moderately thick, like a thick milkshake or smoothie. Such moderately thick liquids are difficult to suck through a straw, like a very thick milkshake, or drip off your spoon slowly drop by drop when you turn it upside down, such as honey.

D.   Circle this if your liquids are very thick, like pudding. Such very thick liquids will stick to a spoon when you turn it upside down, such as pudding.

E.   Circle this if you did not take any liquids by mouth or if you have been limited to ice chips.

13.   In general, would you say your health is:

(circle one)

Poor 1

Fair.. 2

Good 3

Very Good.. 4

Excellent 5

General Questions About You

What is the date of your birth?

Please write in your date of birth here: _____/_____/_____
month   day   year

What is your age today? _____

Are you –

(circle one)

Male 1

Female 2

What is your <u>main</u> racial or ethnic group?

(circle one)

White or Caucasian, but not Hispanic or Latino......................... 1

Black or African-American, but not Hispanic or Latino................ 2

Hispanic or Latino 3

Asian 4

Other 5

What is the highest year of school or college you have ever completed?

(circle one number)

1	2	3	4	5	6	7	8	9	10	11	12	13	14	15	16	16+
Grade School								High School				College				Post Graduate

215

What is your current marital status?

(circle one)

Never married 1

Married... 2

Divorced... 3

Separated 4

Widowed 5

Did anybody help you complete this questionnaire?

(circle one)

No, I did it myself... 1

Yes, someone helped me fill it out... 2

IF SOMEONE HELPED YOU FILL OUT THIS QUESTIONNAIRE, how did that person help you?

(circle one)

Read you the questions and/or wrote down the answers you gave 1

Answered the questions for you 2

Helped in some other way 3

Please write today's date here: _____/_____/_____
                                 month   day   year

Last Page

COMMENTS:

Do you have any comments about this questionnaire? We welcome your comments about the questionnaire in general or about specific questions, especially any that were unclear or confusing to you.

_____

_____

_____

_____

_____

_____

_____

Thank you for completing this questionnaire!

Note: Reprinted with permission of Collen McHorney. For additional information, see McHorney, C. A., Bricker, D. E., Kramer, A. E, Rosenbek, J. C., Robbins, J., Chignell, K. A., et al. (2000). The SWAL-QOL outcomes tool for oropharyngeal dysphagia in adults: I. Conceptual foundation and item development. *Dysphagia*, 15, 115-121; McHorney, C. A., Bricker, D. E., Robbins, J., Kramer, A. E., Rosenbek, J. C., & Chignell, K. A. (2000). The SWAL-QOL outcomes tool for oropharyngeal dysphagia in adults: II. Item reduction and preliminary scaling. *Dysphagia*, 15, 122-133; McHorney, C. A., Martin-Harris, B., Robbins, J., & Rosenbek, J. (2006). Clinical validity of the SWAL-QOL and SWAL-CARE outcome tools with respect to bolus flow measures. *Dysphagia*, 21, 141-148; McHorney, C. A., Robbins, J., Lomax, K., Rosenbek, J. C., Chignell, K. A., Kramer, A. E., et al. (2002). The SWAL-QOL and SWAL-CARE outcomes tool for oropharyngeal dysphagia in adults: III. Documentation of reliability and validity. *Dysphagia*, 17, 97-114.

Appendix B

The Penetration-Aspiration Scale (PAS)

Score	Description
1	No material enters the airway.
2	Material enters the larynx, remains above the folds and is ejected.
3	Material enters the airway, remains above the folds and is not ejected.
4	Material enters the larynx to the level of the vocal folds but is ejected.
5	Material enters the larynx to the level of the folds and is not ejected.
6	Material passes below the vocal folds but is ejected into the larynx or pharynx.
7	Material passes below the vocal folds but is not ejected despite effort.
8	Material passes below the vocal folds with no response from the person (silent aspiration).

Note. From "A Penetration-Aspiration Scale," by J. C. Rosenbek, J. A. Robbins, E. B. Roecker, J. L. Coyle, and J. L. Wood, 1996, *Dysphagia, 11*, pp. 93–98. Republished with permission of Springer Science and Business Media.

Appendix C

Apathy Evaluation Scale[1]

The Apathy Evaluation Scale (AES) was developed to provide global measures of apathy in adults and elderly individuals.[2] Reliability and validity data are available for middle-aged and older adults (2). Examination of individual items also provides qualitative information, which may be of use in clinical assessments. The conceptual, clinical, and empirical background for the AES is presented in several publications (2–7). This background, along with descriptions of other applications of apathy and the AES, is summarized in more recent work (8–10). Essential aspects of this background are presented here as an introduction to the use of the AES.

Detecting apathy depends on identifying specific changes in 3 areas: observable (overt) activity, thought content, and emotional responsivity.

Decrements in overt behavior may entail subtle inefficiencies in the way people get their work done at home or at work. Or they may entail severe impairments in initiating and sustaining goal-directed behavior such that patients require prompting to perform personal and instrumental activities of daily living.

The cognition of patients with apathy reveals a decrease in goal-related thought content. For example, patients will report, "I have no plans," "I'm just not interested in much any more," or "I have little desire to do anything today."

Diminished emotional responsivity refers to shallow, abbreviated, or unchanging emotion in response to goal-related events. For example, confronted with personal losses, health problems, or financial misfortune, patients with apathy will be described as emotionally indifferent, placid, inappropriately euphoric, or affectively shallow or flat. Favorable events similarly elicit attenuated emotional responses.

There are many explanations for symptoms such as these. Diminished activity, diminished goals, and attenuated emotional responses occur in many psychiatric, neurological, and medical disorders (3, 8). What distinguishes apathy is that all three aspects of goal-directed behavior—overt activity per se; cognitions associated with goals, such as plans,

---

[1] The Apathy Evaluation Scale was developed by Robert S. Marin, M.D. Development and validation studies are described in Marin, R. S., Biedrzycki R. C., & Firinciogullari, S., Reliability and Validity of the Apathy Evaluation Scale, Psychiatry Research, 38, 143–162, 1991. Published with the permission of Robert S. Marin.

[2] Reliability and validity of a Children's Motivation Scale, based on the AES, has been reported (1).

curiosity, or interests; and emotional responses to goal-related events—are affected simultaneously.

This analysis provides an *operational definition of apathy: simultaneous diminution in the overt behavioral, cognitive, and emotional concomitants of goal-directed behavior.*

The Operational Definition Implies that the Essential Meaning of Apathy Is Lack of Motivation

The critical aspect of this operational definition is that patients with apathy show changes in the behavioral, cognitive, and emotional aspects of *goal-directed behavior*. It is apathy's relationship to goal-directed behavior that implies its essential meaning is lack of motivation. As described by Atkinson (11), motivation is concerned with understanding the "direction, intensity, and persistence" of goal-directed behavior. Or, as summarized by Jones (12), *motivation is concerned with how behavior "gets started, is energized, is sustained, is directed, is stopped and what kind of subjective reaction is present in the organism when all this is going on."* If applied to measuring the severity of apathy these definitions mean that *patients show apathy to the extent that they show diminished activity due to lack of motivation* (relative to the norms for their age and culture) (8). This distinguishes apathy from other causes of diminished activity, such as mood disturbance (depression or anxiety), intel-

lectual capacity (dementia), or attention (delirium).

It is important to realize that, thus identified, patients with apathy are showing diminution in a fundamental aspect of behavior. Western intellectual traditions (13) recognize three realms of behavior: the intellectual, the emotional, and the conative (13).[2] Psychiatric nosology offers many examples of disorders of intellect and emotion. Apathy and related disorders of diminished motivation (8–10) are examples of a third domain of psychopathology defined by impairment in motivation.

Motivation is essential for human adaptation. Therefore, patients with apathy suffer from an impairment which causes disability in virtually all essential areas of human functioning. Diminished motivation increases the risk of treatment failure because patients will not initiate or persist in following prescribed treatments (6, 8). Medication compliance will suffer. Appointments will be missed. Engagement in intensive treatment programs—for example, socialization, physical rehabilitation, vocational training, pulmonary therapy, renal dialysis—will be attenuated.

In summary, apathy means lack of motivation. Motivation or its inverse, apathy, is operationalized in the AES by evaluating the overt behavioral, cognitive, and emotional aspects of goal-directed behavior. Thus, the AES includes items to evaluate: diminished goal-directed overt behavior, for example, diminished productivity, lack of effort, and initiative; cognitive evidence of apathy, for example, lack of interests, lack of curiosity,

---

[2]Conation refers to willed behavior. This is roughly equated with the domain of motivation. The essential difference is that motivation refers to both conscious and unconscious determinants of behavior.

and decrease in the importance attributed to age-appropriate goals or values, e.g., health, finances, or the welfare of others); and emotional evidence of apathy, for example, shallow affect, emotional indifference, and impersistence of emotional responses.

ADMINISTRATION OF THE APATHY EVALUATION SCALE

General Considerations

Three Versions of the AES

The foregoing definitions are incorporated into the AES. The AES is an 18-item scale. It requires 10–20 minutes to administer depending on the subject's abilities and the version used. There are 3 versions of the scale: *self (AES-S)*, *informant (AES-I*; significant other, e.g., personal or professional caregiver), and *clinician (AES-C)* rated versions. This affords flexibility in rating apathy since the clinical population and clinical circumstances often dictate a preference for one form of administration over another.[3] The clinician version has somewhat better validity than the informant version. The overall validity of the AES-S is less than the AES-C and AES-I. Therefore, when possible the clinician version is preferred. The AES assessment of apathy is based on subjects' current functioning. For outpatients or patients rated within 34 days of hospital-

ization, the period rated is defined as the previous 4 weeks. Changes necessary for hospitalized and other institutionalized individuals are discussed later.

Types of Items

Each version consists of the same 18 items. Consistent with the operational definition of apathy, there are 3 types of items: each item is primarily an index of overt goal-directed behavior, goal-related cognitions, or goal-related emotional responses. This categorization of items is indicated in the righthand column of the clinician version of the AES-C: B = behavioral item; C = cognitive item; E = emotional item.[4] Items are worded with positive or negative syntax (+ or −); most are positive. The rating of self-evaluation (SE) and quantifiable (Q) items, as denoted in the righthand column of the AES-C, is described below.

Two Types of Administration Procedures

The self and informant rated versions are administered as *paper and pencil tests*. Cognitively impaired patients can provide meaningful responses,[5] particularly if the rater reads the items and records the subject's responses. Experience to date (2) suggests that primary caregivers are sensitive, reliable sources of information about apathy.

The AES-C is administered as a *semistructured interview*. Items are rated

---

[3]Evidence of reliability of validity of each version has been presented and supported by subsequent studies (see 14–17).

[4]The items for initiative (#17) and motivation (#18) are coded as other (O) since they are not readily classified as B, C, or E items. Their inclusion is based on the psychometric data used for scale development.

[5]Meaningful ratings can be obtained in subjects with Mini-mental state scores as low as 10, particularly if they are rated using the AES-C or AES-I.

based on current functioning as evident from the subject's "thoughts, feelings, and actions" during the past 4 weeks.[6] It is crucial to understand that the AES-C ratings are based on the *clinician's assessment* of the patient's self-reports. In other words, except for the self-evaluation (SE) items discussed below, the *ratings given for the AES-C are based on the clinician's best judgment (or "objective" assessment) of the subject's motivational state*. To carry out this assessment, *verbal and nonverbal data must be evaluated*. Specific Instructions (below) describes how to integrate verbal and nonverbal observations. Two principles underlie the use of nonverbal information: first, as indicated in the above definitions of apathy and motivation, *emotional responsivity provides information about motivational state*; second, *how the individual deals with questions (verbally and nonverbally) is assumed to provide information about how other activities are dealt with* (for example, with initiative, exuberance, or lethargy). Thus, the AES-C interview is viewed, in effect, as a "motivational laboratory": what the subject says and how it's said provides a valid sample of subject's overall motivation in other situations.

Learning to Use the AES

Basic clinical skills suffice to apply the above definitions to administering the AES. The detailed instructions that follow likely will seem complex on first exposure. With minimal experience, however, they are readily appreciated and applied. Before attempting to assimilate the detailed instructions it is recommended that a new user read the sections titled Specific Instructions and the introduction section of Guidelines for Coding Severity. Then administer the scale to 1 or 2 individuals showing minimal and moderately severe levels of apathy. If unfamiliar with the syndrome of apathy (4, 8), it is better to begin with neurological patients who present lack of motivation without depression; patients with Alzheimer's disease of mild to moderate severity often fulfill this requirement. After this brief experience with the AES, the utility of the additional material is readily assimilated.

With modest experience, it will be evident that the AES is based on what is in many ways a common sense clinical approach to interpreting motivation. In the author's experience, bachelor's level raters can be introduced to the concept of apathy and taught to use the AES with adequate reliability with only 46 hours' experience. Research levels of interrater agreement can be reached by experienced clinicians by rating as few as 510 subjects.

Specific Instructions

The AES should be administrated in a quiet room. A few minutes should be provided to introduce the scale and its purpose and to develop adequate rapport with the patient to insure satisfactory candor.

---

[6]This information can be supplemented by other clinical information when the rater judges the subject's responses of doubtful validity. In practice this is rarely necessary. For clinical purposes the use of external information presumably enhances the validity of AES-C ratings. However, the impact of this procedure on AES scores has not been evaluated.

A consistent format should be used in introducing the scale and administering the items. The following statement is recommended as an introduction to the procedure. It orients the subject to the domains of interest and provides the rater with an initial database that will be used in rating individual items, in particular, Are you interested in things? (#1): "I am going to ask you a series of questions about your thoughts, feelings, and activities. Base your answers on the last 4 weeks. To begin, tell me about your current interests. Tell me about anything that is of interest to you. For example, hobbies or work; activities you are involved in or that you would like to do; interests within the home or outside; with other people or alone; interests that you may be unable to pursue, but which are of interest to you—for example, swimming even though it's winter or reading even though your vision may not be good enough."

The responses to the first question are carefully observed and recorded. The interviewer should make note of: (1) Number of interests reported; (2) degree of detail reported for each interest; (3) affective aspects of expression (verbal and nonverbal).

The interviewer then states: "Now I'd like you to tell me about your average day. Start from the time you wake up and go to the time you go to sleep."

The interviewer again notes the number of activities, degree of detail, intensity and duration of involvement in activities, and the affect associated with presentation of this information.

To assure consistency in presentation, prompting is indicated only if the subject seems not to understand what information is being sought or has forgotten the question.

Each item of the AES is now presented using the wording of the item itself. Begin with items #1 and #2 even though the information just gathered permits a preliminary evaluation. Additional information may be requested to clarify ambiguous responses, but patients should not be pressed for detail if their initial responses are clear. Simple bridges between items may be used to preserve a conversational quality to the interview. Since AES-C ratings are based on the rater's integration of all verbal and nonverbal information obtained from interviewing the patient, the rating of each item is also influenced by information accumulated through responses to all previous questions. For example, individuals with high standards and high motivation are likely to "expect too much from themselves." This will be increasingly evident over the course of the interview. They may underrate their motivation. Thus, if the subject responds to the final question (Do you have motivation?) with "Somewhat motivated," the rater would record "A Lot," which says, in effect, "She says 'somewhat' just because her standards are so high. Relative to others, her rating is really 'A Lot.'"

Guidelines for Coding Severity

Introduction

The 3 versions of the AES use a similar 4-point, Likert-type scale, "Not at all," "Slightly," "Somewhat," and "A Lot." Criteria for these options are not specified for the AES-S and AES-I. For the AES-C, these four response options are defined as follows:

1. Not at all characteristic (none, no examples given)

2. Slightly characteristic (trivial, questionable, minimal)

> Example: "I guess so." "Yea, sort of." "May be a little."

3. Somewhat characteristic (moderate, definite)

> Example: "Yes." "Definitely." "I enjoy playing bridge and dancing." "A fair amount." (stated without facial or vocal change to suggest intensity)

4. A lot characteristic (a great deal, strongly); "A Lot" requires verbal or nonverbal evidence of intensity

> Example: "Oh yes, absolutely, I love it." "You bet!"

Or nonverbal evidence of intensity such as vigorous head nodding; raising amplitude or frequency of speech; sitting up straight and gesturing with hands, etc.

How much is A Lot? In the AES-C "A lot" refers to a level of activity, interest, or emotional intensity seen in normal individuals. It does not refer to levels of intensity that are "supernormal," e.g., hypomanic or manic. In the AES, manic behavior would be coded as "A Lot" and thus could not be distinguished from a well-functioning normal individual.

Quantifiable (Q) Items

The criteria for applying these codes are quantified for several items (#1, #2, #4, #5, #12). These quantifiable items (labeled Q in right-hand column of AES-C) are rated by counting the number of instances cited by the subject for a particular item (e.g., number of interests, number of friends):

1. Not all characteristic: 0 items
2. Slightly characteristic: 1-2 items

3. Somewhat characteristic: 2-3 items
4. A Lot: 3 or more

Example of rating quantifiable (Q) items:

> Rater: Are you interested in things? (#1)
>
> Subj.: Yes, for sure . . . no question about it.

Comment: "For sure" and "no question" suggest higher levels of intensity, and therefore a rating of 4. A Lot. However, for a quantifiable (Q) item, further information is necessary. Therefore, rater asks:

> Rater: Can you give any examples?
>
> Subj.: Well, sure. I like to keep busy. I'm interested in the house most of the time . . . I have to clean up the house every day . . . maybe read some magazines . . . I guess that's about it.

Comment: Subject identifies only two interests: house care and reading magazines. Therefore, despite initial response, score is 3. Somewhat characteristic.

Guidelines for Evaluating Responses that Fall on the Boundary between Two Response Options

It is common for subjects to provide responses that are on the boundary between two scoring options. For example, in the above example, if the subject also had specified a third interest, such as "We try to go bowling once or twice a week," then there would be a total of 3 responses; these 3 responses could be coded as either Somewhat or A Lot, since 2-3 items merits a Somewhat score and 3 or more is scored

A Lot. The following guidelines are used for such boundary cases:

1. Consider the presence of verbal and nonverbal evidence of affect. In the present example, the initial expressions, "Yea, for sure," and "You bet," suggest higher levels of motivation. This would shift the response to this item to a 4. A Lot. Blunted affect or lack of enthusiasm would suggest a more apathetic scoring and therefore a coding of 3. Somewhat.

2. Consider the degree of differentiation of responses. For example, in rating Item 1 "Interested in things": Score Slightly if a subject simply specifies "reading" (i.e., 1 interest), but Somewhat if 2–3 specific books or television programs can be specified. Similarly, if a subject is interested "only" in reading, but provides multiple examples of reading materials, rate Slightly, Somewhat, or A Lot based on the number of examples given. When subjects offer broad categories such as reading or television, it is appropriate to prompt them once for each item with the question, "Can you give me any examples?"

3. In ambiguous instances, rate toward the more apathetic score.

4. When still in doubt, one may ask the patient whether, for example, "Somewhat" or "A Lot" is the more appropriate descriptor.

Self-Evaluation (SE) Items

The self-evaluation (SE) items (#3, #8, #13, #16) are *coded exclusively on the subject's rating of severity. The clinician rater's appraisal is not considered for SE items.* Thus, if a subject says "A Lot" when asked "Is getting together with friends important to you?" (#12) then the response is coded 4. A Lot—even if the rater's "objective" assessment is 2. Slightly because the subject was able to name only 1 friend in the previous question. The purpose of relying on the subject's self-evaluation is that it indicates that the subject still treats having friends or getting things done during the day (#16), etc. as being very important. In effect, then, SE items are indices of the subjective importance an activity or goal has for the subject. Practically speaking, the SE items are often sensitive to the preservation of motivation in individuals who otherwise seem quite apathetic. Thus, someone who gets little or nothing done each day may still show intact goals or values by asserting that Getting together with friends is "very, (i.e., A lot) important to me."

Using Nonverbal Information to Simplify the Rating of Items 7 and 14

Other than quantifiable and self-evaluation items, the rating given for items is based on the descriptors given above, e.g., 2. Slightly is equivalent to trivial, minimal, or questionable. In practice, these descriptors are sufficient to provide excellent reliability for the AES-C. For two items, additional clarification is helpful for distinguishing between Somewhat and A Lot. These items are 7. S/he approaches life with intensity, and 14. When something good happens, s/he gets excited. For these items, it is recommended that the score is "3. Somewhat characteristic" if the patient affirms that these statements are true without verbal or nonverbal evidence of positive affect and "4. A Lot Characteristic" if such evidence is present. Rating these items is also aided by remembering that the subject's overall level of responding during the rating procedure provides much information regarding how they respond "when something good happens" or whether they "approach life with intensity."

Item #15

Item 15, which concerns an "Accurate understanding of his/her problems," calls on the rater to evaluate the adequacy of patients' insight into their personal or, if present, clinical problems. This item may be introduced by saying, "Now let me ask you this. We've been talking about your interests and activities. But we all have problems too. Could you give me an idea about the things that you view as your problems?" Ratings are then based on the appropriateness and accuracy of the response given.

Scoring the AES

For clinical purposes, apathy is conceptualized as a pathological construct. Therefore, AES items are scored so that high AES scores indicate more apathy, i.e., less motivation. This requires recoding items that are stated with positive (+) or "healthy" syntax. Therefore, all but 3 AES items (#6, #10, #11) have to be recoded. The recoding rules are the same for the AES-S, AES-I, and AES-C. Recoding means changing item codes so that $1 = 4$, $2 = 3$, $3 = 2$, $4 = 1$.

Cutoff Scores

Scores for the AES range from 18 to 72. In the original validation study (12), the mean (standard deviation) score for 30 healthy elderly controls were: AES-C: 26 (+/−6); AES-I: 26 (+/−7.5); AES-S: 28 (+/− 6).

Using a criterion of mean + 2 SD this suggests cutoff scores of 39–41, depending on which version of the AES is used. Clinical correlation suggests that these cutoffs are probably slightly low. This is undoubtedly due at least in part to the effect of "volunteerism": individuals who volunteer for a study on apathy probably have higher than average motivation compared to the general population. It should also be noted that the original validation study was performed in a geriatric population. Age and culture are important sources of variance for rating apathy. Also of importance is that the number of healthy controls (n = 30) was insufficient for a standardization procedure. For these reasons, the author recommends that investigators using the AES develop their own norms.

Clinicians using the AES-C in a sample over age 60 years will find that a score of 42 or more generally indicates minimal or mild apathy. Somewhat lower scores are probably significant in younger populations. However, formal recommendations cannot be given at this time.

Using the AES in Hospitals or Other Institutional Environments

The AES was originally developed for individuals living outside of residential environments, which structure much of individuals' daily behavior, e.g. through treatment programs, group meetings, etc. This approach was taken for strategic purposes. The original study was a construct validation study. Priority was given to eliminating the confounding effect on motivation of evaluating subjects when much of their goal-directed behavior was dictated by the external environment. To adapt the AES for this and other effects of institutionalization a few minor adjustments are needed.

1. Motivational Impact of Change in Environment

Being admitted to a hospital, nursing home, rehabilitation facility, or other institution is expected to alter motivation. This does not indicate a weakness of the AES or the concept of apathy. Rather, it reflects the fact that motivation is determined by an interaction between biological, psychological, *and* socioenvironmental variables. This should be considered in deciding how to administer the AES for people in institutions. The author recommends the following.

a. Items that Refer to Activities which Are Directly Structured by the Environment. As a measure of motivation, the AES is concerned with thoughts, feelings, and actions, which represent the subject's initiative, effort, interests, etc. Therefore, subjects should not be given credit for having initiated an activity which was dictated by the schedule or program of the environment. Therefore, "getting things done during the day," "putting effort into the things that interest you," having initiative, etc. are evaluated relative to activities initiated or carried out by the individual *in addition to those strictly called for by the patient's schedule or treatment plan*. An example is helpful. For the item (#2), "He or she gets things done during the day," a subject does not receive credit for going to the regularly scheduled 10 a.m. group therapy session. But reading a book, playing one's own videogame, or writing a letter in unscheduled time all would. Note that not all AES items are so susceptible to such environmental effects. For example, the response to "getting things done during the day is important to me" is not directly influenced by such environmental effects.

2. Ambiguity in Defining Period of Current Functioning in Subjects Recently Admitted to Hospitals or Other Institutions

The general instructions state that current functioning refers to the 4 weeks prior to the time of evaluation.

a. Individuals who have been hospitalized for only a few days should answer AES questions with reference to the 4 weeks *prior* to their admission. After only a few days, it is easy and usually natural to report one's general level of functioning for the preceding 4 weeks.

b. Once individuals have been hospitalized for a week or more, they should consider "current functioning" as their thoughts, feelings, and actions *within the institution*. When admission occurred less than 4 weeks previously it is generally best to restrict the period of interest to the most recent 1–3 weeks. In other words, once adjusted to a hospital environment, the subject ignores the period prior to hospitalization.

c. Periods as short as 1 week generally permit useful reference periods for evaluating motivational status with the AES. Thus, if there has been an acute event, such as a stroke, or if there has been a marked improvement in functioning, for example, due to successful treatment of apathy or depression, a shorter period —one representing relative stability—is appropriate.

SUMMARY

In summary, the guidelines for the AES-C are:

1. Prime the subject with the two questions regarding current interests and daily activities.
2. Administer each item using the wording of each item.
3. Except for self-evaluation (SE) items, the rater integrates verbal and non-verbal information to rate each item. Responses to items are based on the subject's response to the individual item and other information already acquired during the course of the interview. Self-evaluation items are rated exclusively on the basis of the subject's judgment.
4. Guidelines are provided to distinguish between ratings of Not at all, Slightly, Somewhat, and A Lot characteristic. For quantifiable (Q) items, the number of examples and the degree of differentiation for each example are considered in rating each item.
5. Boundary responses are rated by considering verbal and nonverbal evidence of affect, degree of differentiation of responses, subject's judgment regarding the more appropriate rating category, and by rating toward the more apathetic coding.
6. Additional suggestions are included to help in rating Items 7, 14, and 15.
7. Minor adjustments are helpful in rating individuals recently hospitalized or residing in institutions.

Additional questions, comments, or suggestions are welcome. Refer them to Robert S. Marin, M.D., Western Psychiatric Institute and Clinic, 3811 O'Hara St., Pittsburgh, PA 15213. Tel. 412 586 9305. E-mail: marinr@upmc.edu

REFERENCES

1. Gerring JP, Freund L, Gerson, AC, Joshi, PT, et al: Psychometric characteristics of the Children's Motivation Scale. [Peer Reviewed Journal] Psychiatry Research Vol 63(2-3) Jul 1996, 205-217. Elsevier Science, United Kingdom.
2. Marin RS, Biedrzycki RC, Firinciogullari S: Reliability and validity of the Apathy Evaluation Scale. Psychiatry Res 38: 143-162, 1991.
3. Marin RS: Differential diagnosis and classification of apathy. Am J Psychiatry 147:22-30, 1990.
4. Marin RS: Apathy: A neuropsychiatric syndrome. J Neuropsych Clin Neurosci 3:243-254, 1991.
5. Marin RS Firinciogullari S, Biedrzycki RC: The sources of convergence between measures of apathy and depression. J Affective Disorders 28:117-124, 1993.
6. Marin RS, Fogel BS, Hawkins J, et al : Apathy: A treatable syndrome. J Neuropsychiatry and Clinical Neurosciences 7: 23-30, 1995.
7. Marin RS, Firinciogullari MS, Biedrzycki RC: Group differences in the relationship between apathy and depression. J Nerv Ment Dis 182:235-239, 1994.
8. Marin RS: Apathy and related disorders of diminished motivation, in Dickstein LJ, Riba MB, Oldham JM (eds): American Psychiatric Association Review of Psychiatry Vol 15. Washington, DC, American Psychiatric Press, Inc., 1996.
9. Marin RS: Apathy: Concept, syndrome, neural mechanisms and treatment. Seminars in Neuropsychiatry (in press).
10. Duffy JD, Marin RS: Issue devoted "Apathy and related disorders of diminished motivation." Psychiatric Annals (in press).

11. Atkinson, JW, Birch, D: An Introduction to Motivation. Princeton, NJ, Van Nostrand, 1978

12. Jones MR: Introduction. In Jones MR (ed), Nebraska Symposium on Motivation. p v x, Lincoln University of Nebraska Press, 195513. Hillgard ER: The trilogy of mind: cognition, affection and conation. J Hist Behav Sci 16:107–117, 1980.

14. Starkstein SE, Mayberg HS, Preziosi TJ, et al: Reliability, validity, and clinical correlates of apathy in Parkinson's disease. Journal of Neuropsychiatry and Clinical Neurosciences, 4:134–139, 1992.

15. Starkstein SE, Federoff JP, Price TR, et al: Apathy following cerebrovascular lesions. Stroke 24:1625–1630, 1993.

16. Kant R, Duffy JD, Pivovarnik A: The prevalence of apathy following closed head injury. Journal Neuropsychiatry and Clinical Neurosciences, 7:425(A) 1996.

Apathy Evaluation Scale (Clinician Version)

Name: _____   Date: ____/____/____

Rater: _____

Rate each item based on an interview of the subject. The interview should begin with a description of the subject's interests, activities, and daily routine. Base your ratings on both verbal and nonverbal information. Ratings should be based on the past 4 weeks. For each item ratings should be judged:

Not at All Characteristic	Slightly Characteristic	Somewhat Characteristic	A Lot Characteristic
1	2	3	4

___ 1. S/he is interested in things.   + C Q*

___ 2. S/he gets things done during the day.   + B Q

___ 3. Getting things started on his/her own is important to him/her.   + C SE

___ 4. S/he is interested in having new experiences.   + C Q

___ 5. S/he is interested in learning new things.   + C Q

___ 6. S/he puts little effort into anything.   – B

___ 7. S/he approaches life with intensity.   + E

___ 8. Seeing a job through to the end is important to her/him.   + C SE

___ 9. S/he spends time doing things that interest her/him.   + B

___ 10. Someone has to tell her/him what to do each day.   – B

___ 11. S/he is less concerned about her/his problems than s/he should be.   – C

___ 12. S/he has friends.   + B Q

___ 13. Getting together with friends is important to him/her.   + C SE

___ 14. When something good happens, s/he gets excited.   + E

___ 15. S/he has an accurate understanding of her/his problems.   + 0

___ 16. Getting things done during the day is important to her/him.   + C SE

___ 17. S/he has initiative.   + 0

___ 18. S/he has motivation.   + 0

The Apathy Evaluation Scale was developed by Robert S. Marin, M.D. Development and validation studies are described in Marin, R. S., Biedrzycki R. C., & Firinciogullari, S., Reliability and Validity of the Apathy Evaluation Scale, *Psychiatry Research*, *38*, 143–162, 1991.

*Note. Items that have positive versus negative syntax are identified by +/–. Type of item: C = cognitive; B = behavior; E = emotional; 0 = other. The definitions of self-evaluation (SE) items and quantifiable items (Q) are discussed in the administrations guidelines (3).

Apathy Evaluation Scale (Informant—Female)

Name: _____ Date: ____/____/____

Informant's Name: _____ Relationship: _____

For each statement, circle the answer that best describes the subject's thoughts, feelings, and activity in the past 4 weeks.

1. She is interested in things.
   NOT AT ALL   SLIGHTLY   SOMEWHAT   A LOT

2. She gets things done during the day.
   NOT AT ALL   SLIGHTLY   SOMEWHAT   A LOT

3. Getting things started on her own is important to her.
   NOT AT ALL   SLIGHTLY   SOMEWHAT   A LOT

4. She is interested in having new experiences.
   NOT AT ALL   SLIGHTLY   SOMEWHAT   A LOT

5. She is interested in learning new things.
   NOT AT ALL   SLIGHTLY   SOMEWHAT   A LOT

6. She puts little effort into anything.
   NOT AT ALL   SLIGHTLY   SOMEWHAT   A LOT

7. She approaches life with intensity.
   NOT AT ALL   SLIGHTLY   SOMEWHAT   A LOT

8. Seeing a job through to the end is important to her.
   NOT AT ALL   SLIGHTLY   SOMEWHAT   A LOT

9. She spends time doing things that interest her.
   NOT AT ALL   SLIGHTLY   SOMEWHAT   A LOT

10. Someone has to tell her what to do each day.
    NOT AT ALL   SLIGHTLY   SOMEWHAT   A LOT

11. She is less concerned about her problems than she should be.
    NOT AT ALL   SLIGHTLY   SOMEWHAT   A LOT

12. She has friends.
    NOT AT ALL   SLIGHTLY   SOMEWHAT   A LOT

13. Getting together with friends is important to her.
    NOT AT ALL   SLIGHTLY   SOMEWHAT   A LOT

continues

14. When something good happens, she gets excited.

     NOT AT ALL   SLIGHTLY   SOMEWHAT   A LOT

15. She has an accurate understanding of her problems.

     NOT AT ALL   SLIGHTLY   SOMEWHAT   A LOT

16. Getting things done during the day is important to her.

     NOT AT ALL   SLIGHTLY   SOMEWHAT   A LOT

17. She has initiative.

     NOT AT ALL   SLIGHTLY   SOMEWHAT   A LOT

18. She has motivation.

     NOT AT ALL   SLIGHTLY   SOMEWHAT   A LOT

The Apathy Evaluation Scale was developed by Robert S. Marin, M.D. Development and validation studies are described in RS Marin, RC Biedrzycki, S Firinciogullari: "Reliability and Validity of the Apathy Evaluation Scale," Psychiatry Research, 38:143–162, 1991.

Apathy Evaluation Scale (Informant—Male)

Name: _____ Date: ____/____/____

Informant's Name: _____ Relationship: _____

For each statement, circle the answer that best describes the subject's thoughts, feelings, and activity in the past 4 weeks.

1. He is interested in things.
   NOT AT ALL   SLIGHTLY   SOMEWHAT   A LOT

2. He gets things done during the day.
   NOT AT ALL   SLIGHTLY   SOMEWHAT   A LOT

3. Getting things started on his own is important to him.
   NOT AT ALL   SLIGHTLY   SOMEWHAT   A LOT

4. He is interested in having new experiences.
   NOT AT ALL   SLIGHTLY   SOMEWHAT   A LOT

5. He is interested in learning new things.
   NOT AT ALL   SLIGHTLY   SOMEWHAT   A LOT

6. He puts little effort into anything.
   NOT AT ALL   SLIGHTLY   SOMEWHAT   A LOT

7. He approaches life with intensity.
   NOT AT ALL   SLIGHTLY   SOMEWHAT   A LOT

8. Seeing a job through to the end is important to him.
   NOT AT ALL   SLIGHTLY   SOMEWHAT   A LOT

9. He spends time doing things that interest him.
   NOT AT ALL   SLIGHTLY   SOMEWHAT   A LOT

10. Someone has to tell him what to do each day.
    NOT AT ALL   SLIGHTLY   SOMEWHAT   A LOT

11. He is less concerned about his problems than he should be.
    NOT AT ALL   SLIGHTLY   SOMEWHAT   A LOT

12. He has friends.
    NOT AT ALL   SLIGHTLY   SOMEWHAT   A LOT

13. Getting together with friends is important to him.
    NOT AT ALL   SLIGHTLY   SOMEWHAT   A LOT

continues

14. When something good happens, he gets excited.

     NOT AT ALL   SLIGHTLY   SOMEWHAT   A LOT

15. He has an accurate understanding of his problems.

     NOT AT ALL   SLIGHTLY   SOMEWHAT   A LOT

16. Getting things done during the day is important to him.

     NOT AT ALL   SLIGHTLY   SOMEWHAT   A LOT

17. He has initiative.

     NOT AT ALL   SLIGHTLY   SOMEWHAT   A LOT

18. He has motivation.

     NOT AT ALL   SLIGHTLY   SOMEWHAT   A LOT

The Apathy Evaluation Scale was developed by Robert S. Marin, M.D. Development and validation studies are described in RS Marin, RC Biedrzycki, S Firinciogullari: "Reliability and Validity of the Apathy Evaluation Scale," Psychiatry Research, 38: 143–162, 1991.

Apathy Evaluation Scale (Self-Rated)

Name: _____   Date: ____/____/____

For each statement, circle the answer that best describes the subject's thoughts, feelings, and activity in the past 4 weeks.

1. I am interested in things.
   NOT AT ALL   SLIGHTLY   SOMEWHAT   A LOT

2. I get things done during the day.
   NOT AT ALL   SLIGHTLY   SOMEWHAT   A LOT

3. Getting things started on my own is important to me.
   NOT AT ALL   SLIGHTLY   SOMEWHAT   A LOT

4. I am interested in having new experiences.
   NOT AT ALL   SLIGHTLY   SOMEWHAT   A LOT

5. I am interested in learning new things.
   NOT AT ALL   SLIGHTLY   SOMEWHAT   A LOT

6. I put little effort into anything.
   NOT AT ALL   SLIGHTLY   SOMEWHAT   A LOT

7. I approach life with intensity.
   NOT AT ALL   SLIGHTLY   SOMEWHAT   A LOT

8. Seeing a job through to the end is important to me.
   NOT AT ALL   SLIGHTLY   SOMEWHAT   A LOT

9. I spend time doing things that interest me.
   NOT AT ALL   SLIGHTLY   SOMEWHAT   A LOT

10. Someone has to tell me what to do each day.
    NOT AT ALL   SLIGHTLY   SOMEWHAT   A LOT

11. I am less concerned about my problems than I should be.
    NOT AT ALL   SLIGHTLY   SOMEWHAT   A LOT

12. I have friends.
    NOT AT ALL   SLIGHTLY   SOMEWHAT   A LOT

13. Getting together with friends is important to me.
    NOT AT ALL   SLIGHTLY   SOMEWHAT   A LOT

continues

14. When something good happens, I get excited.

  NOT AT ALL   SLIGHTLY   SOMEWHAT   A LOT

15. I have an accurate understanding of my problems.

  NOT AT ALL   SLIGHTLY   SOMEWHAT   A LOT

16. Getting things done during the day is important to me.

  NOT AT ALL   SLIGHTLY   SOMEWHAT   A LOT

17. I have initiative.

  NOT AT ALL   SLIGHTLY   SOMEWHAT   A LOT

18. I have motivation.

  NOT AT ALL   SLIGHTLY   SOMEWHAT   A LOT

The Apathy Evaluation Scale was developed by Robert S. Marin, M.D. Development and validation studies are described in RS Marin, RC Biedrzycki, S Firinciogullari: "Reliability and Validity of the Apathy Evaluation Scale," Psychiatry Research, 38:143–1

References

Abele, M., Burk, K., Schols, L., Schwartz, S., Besenthal, I., Dichgans, J., et al. (2002). The aetiology of sporadic adult-onset ataxia. *Brain, 125*, 961–988.

Adler, C. H., Bansberg, S. F., Hentz, J. G., Ramig, L. O., Buder, E. H., Witt, K., et al. (2004). Botulinum toxin type A for treating voice tremor. *Archives of Neurology, 61*, 1416–1420.

Alfonso, M., Ferdjallah, M., Shaker, R., & Wertsch, J. J. (1998). Electrophysiologic validation of deglutitive UES opening head lift exercise [abstract]. *Gastroenterology, 114*, G2942.

Alfonsi, E., Versino, M., Merlo, I. M., Pacchetti, C., Martignoni, E., Bertino, G., et al. (2007). Electrophysiologic patterns of oral-pharyngeal swallowing in parkinsonian syndromes. *Neurology, 68*, 5835–5890.

Alusi, S. H., Aziz, T. Z., Glickman, S., Jahanshahi, M., Stein, J. F., & Bain, P. G. (2001). Stereotactic lesional surgery for the treatment of tremor in multiple sclerosis: A prospective case-controlled study. *Brain, 124*, 1576–1589.

Asgeirsson, H., Jakobsson, F., Hjaltason, H., Jonsdottir, H. & Sveinbjornsdottir, S. (2006). Prevalence study of primary dystonia in Iceland. *Movement Disorders, 21*, 293–298.

Ashford, J., Frymark, T., McCabe, D., Mullen, R., Musson, N., Smith-Hammond, C., et al. (2008). Evidence-based practice systematic review: Oropharyngeal dysphagia behavioral treatments: Part I. Impact of dysphagia treatment on normal swallow function. Manuscript submitted for publication.

Aviv, J. E., Kim, T., Sacco, R. L., Kaplan, S., Goodheart, K., Diamond, B., et al. (1998). FEESST: A new bedside endoscopic test of the motor and sensory components of swallowing. *Annals of Otology, Rhinology, and Laryngology, 107*, 378–387.

Aviv, J. E., & Murry, T. (2005). *FEEST: Flexible endoscopic evaluation of swallowing with sensory testing.* San Diego, CA: Plural.

Bak, T. H. (2008). Overlap syndromes. In J. R. Hodges (Ed.), *Frontotemporal dementia syndromes* (pp. 80–101). Cambridge, UK: Cambridge University Press.

Balash, Y., & Giladi, N. (2004). Efficacy of pharmacological treatment of dystonia: Evidence-based review including meta-analysis of the effect of botulinum toxin and other cure options. *European Journal of Neurology, 11*, 361–370.

Ben-Shlomo, Y., Wenning, G. K., Tison, F., & Quinn, N. P. (1997). Survival of patients with pathologically proven multiple system strophy: A meta-analysis. *Neurology, 48*, 384–393.

Berciano, J. (1982). Olivopontocerebellar atrophy. *Journal of the Neurological Sciences, 53*, 253–272.

Bergman, H., & Deuschl, G. (2002). Pathophysiology of Parkinson's disease: From clinical neurology to neuroscience and back. *Movement Disorders, 17*, S28–S40.

Bhidayasiri, R., & Tarsy, D. (2007). In M. A. Stacy (Ed.), *Handbook of dystonia* (pp. 301–316). New York: Informa Healthcare USA.

Bilney, B., Morris, M. E., & Perry, A. (2003). Effectiveness of physiotherapy, occupational therapy, and speech pathology for people with Huntington's disease: A systematic review. *Neurorehabilitation and Neural Repair, 17*, 12–24.

Bland, S. T., Humm, J. L., Kozlowski, D. A., Williams, L., Strong, R., Aronowski, J., et al. (1998). Forced overuse of the contralateral forelimb increases infarct volume following a mild, but not a severe, transient cerebral ischemic insult. *Society for Neuroscience Abstracts*, *774*, 1955.

Blumenfeld, L., Hahn, Y., Lepage, A., Leonard, R., & Belafsky, P. C. (2006). Transcutaneous electrical stimulation versus traditional dysphagia therapy: A nonconcurrent cohort study. *Otolaryngology–Head and Neck Surgery*, *135*, 754-757.

Bonelli, R. M., Wenning, G. K., & Kapfhammer, H. P. (2004). Huntington's disease: Present treatments and future therapeutic modalities. *International Clinical Psychopharmacology*, *19*, 51-62.

Bosma. J. F. (1986). Self report of K.J.: Dyskinesia—My constant companion. *Dysphagia*, *1*, 19-22.

Braak, H., Del Tredici, K., Rub, U., de Vos, R. A. I., Jansen Steur, E. N., & Braak, E. (2003). Staging of brain pathology related to sporadic Parkinson's disease. *Neurobiology of Aging*, *24*, 197-211.

Braak, H., Ghebremedhin, E., Rub, U., Bratzke, H., & Del Tredici, K. (2004). Stages in the development of Parkinson's disease-related pathology. *Cell and Tissue Research*, *318*, 121-134.

Braak, H., Muller, C. M., Rub, U., Ackerman, H., Bratzke, H., de Vos, R. A. I., et al. (2006). Pathology associated with sporadic Parkinson's disease—Where does it end? *Journal of Neurotransmission*, *70*, 89-97.

Bulow, M., Olsson, R., & Ekberg, O. (1999). Videomanometric analysis of supraglottic swallow, effortful swallow, and chin tuck in healthy volunteers. *Dysphagia*, *14*, 67-72.

Bulow, M., Olsson, R., & Ekberg, O. (2001). Videomanometric analysis of supraglottic swallow, effortful swallow, and chin tuck in patients with pharyngeal dysfunction. *Dysphagia*, *16*, 190-195.

Bulow, M., Olsson, R., & Ekberg, O. (2002). Supraglottic swallow, effortful swallow, and chin tuck did not alter hypopharyngeal intrabolus pressure in patients with pharyngeal dysfunction. *Dysphagia*, *17*, 197-201,

Burk, K., Abele, M., Fetter, M., Dichgans, J., Skalej, M., Laccone, F., et al. (1996). Autosomal dominant cerebellar ataxia type I: Clinical features and MRI in families with SCA1, SCA2 and SCA3. *Brain*, *119*, 1497-1505.

Burke, R., Fahn, S., Marsden, C., Bressman, S., Mokowitz, C., & Friedman, J. (1985). Validity and reliability of a rating scale for the primary torsion dystonias. *Neurology*, *35*, 73-77.

Bushmann, M., Dobmeyer, S. M., Leeker, L., & Perlmutter, J. S. (1989). Swallowing abnormalities and their response to treatment in Parkinson's disease. *Neurology*, *39*, 1309-1314.

Butler, A. G., Duffey, P. O., Hawthorne, M. R., & Barnes, M. P. (2004). An epidemiologic survey of dystonia within the entire population of northeast England over the past nine years. *Advances in Neurology*, *94*, 95-99.

Carnaby-Mann, G. D., & Crary, M. (2007). Examining the evidence on neuromuscular stimulation for swallowing: A meta-analysis. *Archives of Otolaryngology–Head & Neck Surgery*, *133*, 564-571.

Caroff, S. N., Mann, S. C., Campbell, E. C., & Sullivan, K. A. (2002). Movement disorders associated with atypical antipsychotic drugs. *Journal of Clinical Psychiatry*, *63*, 12-19.

Castell, J. A., Castell, D. O., Schultz, A. R., & Georgeson, S. (1993). Effect of head position on the dynamics of the upper esophageal sphincter and pharynx. *Dysphagia*, *14*, 1-6.

Cersosimo, M. G., Juri, S., Suárez de Chandler, S., Clerici, R., & Micheli, F. E. (2005). Swallowing dysfunction in patients with blepharospasm. *Medicina (Beunos Aires)*, *65*, 117-120.

Cersosimo, M. G, & Koller, W. C. (2004). Essential tremor. In R. L. Watts & W. C.

Koller (Eds.), *Movement disorders: Neurologic principles and practice* (2nd ed.) (pp. 431–458). New York: McGraw-Hill.

Cersosimo, M. G., Raina, G. B., Piedimonte, F., Antico, J., Graff, P., & Micheli, F. E. (2008). Pallidal surgery for the treatment of primary generalized dystonia: Long-term follow-up. *Clinical Neurology and Neurosurgery, 110*, 145–150.

Colodny, N. (2002). Interjudge and intrajudge reliabilities in fiberoptic endoscopic evaluation of swallowing (FEES®) using the Penetration-Aspiration Scale: A replication study. *Dysphagia, 17*, 308–315.

Comella, C. L., Jankovic, J., Shannon, K. M., Swenson, M., Leurgans, S., Fan, W., et al. (2005). Comparison of botulinum toxin serotypes A and B for the treatment of cervical dystonia. *Neurology, 65*, 1423–1429.

Comella, C. L., Leurgans, S., Wuu, J., Stebbins, G. T., Chmura, T., & the Dystonia Study Group. (2003). Rating scales for dystonia: A multicenter assessment. *Movement Disorders, 18*, 303–312.

Consky, E., Basinki, A., Belle, L., Ranawaya, R., & Lang, A. (1990). The Toronto Western Spasmodic Torticollis Rating Scale (TWSTRS): Assessment of validity and interrater reliability. *Neurology, 40*, 445.

Corbin-Lewis, K., Liss, J. M., & Sciortino, K. L. (2005). Clinical anatomy & physiology of the swallow mechanism. Clifton Park, NY: Thomson Delmar Learning.

Countryman, S., & Ramig, L. O. (1994). Speech and voice deficits in Parkinsonian plus syndromes: Can they be treated? *Journal of Medical Speech-Language Pathology, 2*, 211–225

Crary, M. A. (1995). A direct intervention program for chronic neurogenic dysphagia secondary to brainstem stroke. *Dysphagia, 10*, 6–18.

Crary, M. A., Carnaby-Mann, G. D., & Faunce, A. (2007). Electrical stimulation therapy for dysphagia: Descriptive results of two surveys. *Dysphagia, 22*, 165–173.

Crary, M. A., Carnaby-Mann, G. D., & Groher, M. E. (2004). Functional benefits of dys-phagia therapy using adjunctive sEMG biofeedback. *Dysphagia, 19*, 160–164.

Da Silva-Junior, F. P., Carrasco, A. E., da Silva Mendes, A. M., Lopes, A. J., Nobre E Souza, M. A., & de Bruin, V. M. (2007). Swallowing dysfunction in Wilson's disease: A scintigraphic study. *Neurogastroenterology Motility, 20*, 285–290.

Dauer, W. T., Burke, R. E., Greene, P., & Fahn, S. (1998). Current concepts on the clinical features, aetiology and management of idiopathic cervical dystonia. *Brain, 121*, 547–560.

David, G., Durr, A., Stevanin, G., Cancel, G., Abbas, N., Benomar, A., et al. (1998). Molecular and clinical correlations in autosomal dominant cerebellar ataxia with progressive macular dystrophy (SCA7). *Human Molecular Genetics, 7*, 165–170.

The Deep-Brain Stimulation for Parkinson's Disease Study Group. (2001). Deep-brain stimulation of the subthalamic nucleus or the pars interna of the globus pallidus in Parkinson's disease. *New England Journal of Medicine, 345*, 956–963.

Defazio, G. (2007). Epidemiology of primary and secondary dystonia. In M. A. Stacy (Ed.), *Handbook of dystonia* (pp. 11–20). New York: Informa Healthcare USA.

De Rijk, M. C., Tzourio, C., Breteler, M. M., Dartigues, J. F., Amaducci, L., Lopez-Pousa, S., et al. (1997). Prevalence of parkinsonism and Parkinson's disease in Europe: The EUROPARKINSON Collaborative study. European Concerted Action on the Epidemiology of Parkinson's disease. *Journal of Neurology, Neurosurgery, and Psychiatry, 62*, 10–15.

Dickson, D. W., Bergeron, C., Chin, S. S., Duyckaerts, C., Horoupian, D., Ikeda, K., et al. (2002). Office of rare diseases neuropathologic criteria for corticobasal degeneration. *Journal of Neuropathology and Experimental Neurology, 61*, 935–946.

Diroma, C., Dell'Aquila, C., Fraddosion, A., Lamberti, S., Mastronardi, R., Russo, I., et al. (2003). Natural history and clinical features of progressive supranuclear palsy:

A clinical study. *Neurological Sciences*, *24*, 176-177.

Duane, D. D. (1988). Spasmodic torticollis: Clinical and biologic features and their implications for focal dystonia. *Advances in Neurology*, *49*, 135-150.

Dung Le, K., Niulsen, B., & Dietrichs, E. (2003). Prevalence of primary focal and segmental dystonia in Oslo. *Neurology*, *61*, 1294-1296.

Durif, F., Lemaire, J. J., Debilly, B., & Dordian, G. (2002). Long-term follow-up of globus pallidus chronic stimulation in advanced Parkinson's disease. *Movement Disorders*, *17*, 803-807.

Elia, A. E., Filippini, G., Bentivoglio, A. R., Fasano, A., Ialongo, T., & Albanese, A. (2006). Onset and progression of primary torsion dystonia in sporadic and familial cases. *European Journal of Neurology*, *13*, 1083-1088.

El Sharkawi, A., Ramig, L., Logemann, J., Pauloski, B. R., Rademaker, A. W., Smith, C. H., et al. (2002). Swallowing and voice effects of Lee Silverman Voice Treatment (LSVT): A pilot study. *Journal of Neurology, Neurosurgery, and Psychiatry*, *72*, 31-36.

Ertekin, C. (2002). Physiological and pathological aspects of oropharyngeal swallowing. *Movement disorders*, *17*(Suppl. 2), S86-S89.

Ertekin, C., Keskin, A., Niylioglu, N., Kirazli, Y., On, A. Y., Tarlaci, S., et al. (2001). The effect of head and neck positions on oropharyngeal swallowing: A clinical and electrophysiologic study. *Archives of Physical Medicine and Rehabilitation*, *82*, 1255-1260.

Fahn, S., Bressman, S., & Marsden, C. D. (1998). Classification of dystonia. *Advances in Neurology*, *78*, 1-10.

Fahn, S., Elton, R. L., & UPDRS program members. (1987). The Unified Parkinson's Disease Rating Scale. In S. Fahn, C. D. Marsden, D. B. Calne, & M. Goldstein (Eds.), *Recent developments in Parkinson's disease* (Vol. 2, pp. 153-163). Florham Park, NJ: Macmillan Healthcare Information.

Fahn, S., Marsden, C. D., & Calne, D. B. (1987). Classification and investigation of dystonia. In C. D. Marsden & C. D. Fahn (Eds.), *Movement Disorders 2*, (pp. 332-358). London: Butterworth.

Farley, B. G., Fox, C. M., Ramig, L. O., & MacFarland, D. (in press). Intensive amplitude-specific therapeutic approaches for Parkinson disease: Toward a neuroplasticity-principled rehabilitation model. *Topics in Geriatric Rehabilitation*.

Fernandez, H. H., Rodriguez, R. L., Skidmore, F. M., & Okun, M. S. (2007). *A practical approach to movement disorders*. New York: Demos Medical.

Feve, A., Angelard, B., Fenelon, G., Logak, M., Guillard, A., & Lacau Saint-Guily, J. (1993). Postneuroleptic laryngeal dyskinesias: A cause of upper airway obstruction syndrome improved by local injections of botulinum toxin. *Movement Disorders*, *8*, 217-219.

Feve, A., Angelard, B., & St Guily, J. L. (1995). Laryngeal tardive dyskinesia. *Journal of Neurology*, *242*, 455-459.

Folstein, M., Folstein, S. E., & McHugh, P. R. (1975). "Mini-Mental State." A practical method for grading the cognitive state of patients for the clinician. *Journal of Psychiatric Research*, *12*, 189-198.

Fraser, C., Power, M., Hamdy, S., Rothwell, J., Hobday, D., Hollander, I., et al. (2002). Driving plasticity in adult human motor cortex is associated with improved motor function after brain injury. *Neuron*, *34*, 831-840.

Frattali, C. M., & Sonies, B. C. (2000). Speech and swallowing disturbances in corticobasal degeneration. In I. Litvan, C. G. Goetz, & A. E. Lang (Eds.), *Advances in Neurology*, *82*, 153-160.

Freed, M. L., Freed, L., Chatburn, R. L., & Christian, M. (2001). Electrical stimulation for swallowing disorders caused by stroke. *Respiratory Care*, *46*, 466-474.

Friedman, J. H. (1998). Rapid onset tardive dyskinesia ("fly catcher tongue") in a neuroleptically naïve patient induced by risperidone. *Medicine and Health, Rhode Island, 81,* 271–272.

Fujiu, M., & Logemann, J. A. (1996). Effect of a tongue-holding maneuver on posterior pharyngeal wall movement during deglutition. *American Journal of Speech-Language Pathology, 5,* 23–30.

Fujiu, M., Logemann, J. A., & Pauloski, B. (1995). Increased post-operative posterior pharyngeal movement in patients with anterior oral cancer: Preliminary finding and possible implications for treatment. *American Journal of Speech-Language Pathology, 4,* 24–30.

Genis, D., Matilla, T., Volpini, V., Rosell, J., Davalos, A., Ferrer, I., et al. (1995). Clinical, neuropathologic, and genetic studies of a large spinocerebellar ataxia type 1 (SCA1) kindred: (CAG)n expansion and early premonitory signs and symptoms. *Neurology, 45,* 24–30.

Gibbons, R. B. (2000). Resolving nutritional challenges of the patient with Parkinson's disease. *Home Healthcare Consultant, 7,* 21–27.

Gilman, S. (2000). The spinocerebellar ataxias. *Clinical Neuropharmacology, 23,* 296–303.

Gilman, S. (2004). Clinical features and treatment of cerebellar disease. In R. L. Watts & W. C. Koller (Eds.), *Movement disorders: Neurologic principles and practice* (2nd ed., pp. 723–736). New York: McGraw-Hill.

Gilman, S., Low, P. A., Quinn, N., Albanese, A., Ben-Shlomo, Y., Fowler, C. J., et al. (1999). Consensus statement on the diagnosis of multiple system atrophy. *Journal of the Neurological Sciences, 163,* 94–98.

Goetz, C. G., & Horn, S. (2004). Tardive dyskinesia. In R. L. Watts & W. C. Koller (Eds.), *Movement disorders: Neurologic principles and practice* (2nd ed., pp. 629–637). New York: McGraw-Hill.

Goetz, C. G., Leurgans, S., Lang, A. E., & Litvan, I. (2003). Progression of gait, speech and swallowing deficits in progressive supranuclear palsy. *Neurology, 60,* 917–922.

Goetz, C. G., Poewe, W., Rascol, O., Sampaio, C., Stebbins, G. T, Counsell, C., et al. (2004).

Movement Disorder Society Task Force report on the Hoehn and Yahr staging scale: Status and recommendations. *Movement Disorders, 19,* 1020–1028.

Golbe, L. I. (1994). The epidemiology of PSP. *Journal of Neural Transmission, 42,* 263–273.

Golbe, L. I. (2004). Progressive supranuclear palsy (Richardson's disease). In R. L. Watts & W. C. Koller (Eds.), *Movement disorders: Neurologic principles and practice* (2nd ed., pp. 339–358). New York: McGraw-Hill.

Golper, L. A. C., Nutt, J. G., Rau, M. T., & Coleman, R. O. (1983). Focal cranial dystonias. *Journal of Speech and Hearing Disorders, 48,* 128–134.

Gouider-Khouja, H., Vidailhet, M., Bonnet, A. M., Pichon, J., & Agid, Y. (1995). "Pure" striatonigral degeneration and Parkinson's disease: A comparative clinical study. *Movement Disorders, 10,* 288–294.

Greene, P., Kang, U. J., & Fahn, F. (1995). Spread of symptoms in idiopathic torsion dystonia. *Movement Disorders, 10,* 143–152.

Gregory, R. P., Smith, P. T., & Rudge, P. (1992). Tardive dyskinesia presenting as severe dysphagia. *Journal of Neurology, Neurosurgery, and Psychiatry, 55,* 1203–1204.

Gulyas, A. E., & Salazar-Grueso, E. F. (1988). Pharyngeal dysmotility in a patient with Wilson's disease. *Dysphagia, 2,* 230–234.

Hamakawa, S., Koda, C., Umeno, H., Yoshida, Y., Nakashima, T., Asoka, K., et al. (2004). Oropharyngeal dysphagia in a case of Huntington's disease. *Auris Nasus Larynx, 31,* 171–176.

Harris, M. L., Julyan, P., Kulkarni, B., Gow, D., Hobson, A., Hastings, D., et al. (2005). Mapping metabolic brain activation during human volitional swallowing: A positron emission tomography study using [18F] fluorodeoxyglucose. *Journal of Cerebral Blood Flow and Metabolism, 25,* 520–526.

Hayashi, T., Nishikawa, T., Koga, I., Uchida, Y., & Yamawaki, S. (1997). Life-threatening dysphagia following prolonged neuroleptic therapy. *Clinical Neuropharmacology, 20,* 77–81.

Hays, N. P., & Roberts, S. B. (2006). The anorexia of aging in adults. *Physiology & Behavior, 88,* 257–266.

Hewitt, A., Hind, J., Kays, S., Nicosia, M., Doyle, J., Tompkins, W., et al. (2008). Standardized instrument for lingual pressure measurement. *Dysphagia, 23,* 16–25.

Higo, R., Nito, T., & Tayama, N. (2005). Swallowing function in patients with multiple-system atrophy with a clinical predominance of cerebellar symptoms (MSA-C). *European Archives of Otolaryngology, 262,* 646–650.

Higo, R., Tayama, N., Watanabe, T., Nitou, T., & Takeuchi, S. (2003a). Vocal fold motion impairment in patients with multiple system atrophy: Evaluation of its relationship with swallowing function. *Journal of Neurology, Neurosurgery, and Psychiatry, 74,* 982–984.

Higo, R., Tayama, N., Watanabe, T., Nitou, T., & Ugawa, Y. (2003b). Videofluoroscopic swallowing function in patients with multiple system atrophy. *Annals of Otology, Rhinology, and Laryngology, 112,* 630–636.

Hind, J. A., Nicosia, M. A., Roecker, E. B., Carnes, M. L., & Robbins, J. (2001). Comparison of effortful and noneffortful swallows in healthy middle-aged and older adults. *Archives of Physical Medicine and Rehabilitation, 82,* 1661-1665.

Hirano, K., Takahashi, K., Uyama, R., Yamashita, Y., Yokoyama, M., Michiwaki, Y., et al. (1999). Objective evaluation of swallow maneuver (Showa swallow maneuver) using CT images. *Dysphagia, 14,* 127.

Hixon, T. J., & Hoit, J. D. (2005). *Evaluation and management of speech breathing disorders: Principles and methods.* Tucson, AZ: Redington Brown.

Hodges, J. R. (2007). *Frontotemporal dementia syndromes.* Cambridge, UK: Cambridge University Press.

Hoehn, M. M., & Yahr, M. D. (1967). Parkinsonism: Onset, progression and mortality. *Neurology, 17,* 427–442.

Holmes, G. (1939). The cerebellum of man: Hughlings Jackson Lecture. *Brain, 62,* 1.

Horner, J., Riski, J. E., Ovelmen-Levitt, J., & Nashold, B. S. (1992). Swallowing in torti-collis before and after rhizotomy. *Dysphagia, 7,* 117–125.

Horner, J., Riski, J. E., Weber, B. A., & Nashold, B. S. (1993). Swallowing, speech, and brainstem auditory-evoked potentials in spasmodic torticollis. *Dysphagia, 8,* 29–34.

Horstink, M., Tolosa, E., Bonuccelli, U., Deuschl, G., Freidman, A., Kanovsky, P., et al. (2006). Review of the therapeutic management of parkinson's disease. Report of a joint task force of the European Federation of the Neurological Societies (EFNS) and the Movement Disorder Society-European Section (MBS-ES). Part I: Early (uncomplicated) parkinson's disease. *European Journal of Neurology, 13,* 1170–1185.

Horstink, M., Tolosa, E., Bonuccelli, U., Deuschl, G., Freidman, A., Kanovsky, P., et al. (2006). Review of the therapeutic management of parkinson's disease. Review of a joint task force of the European Federation of the Neurological Societies (EFNS) and the Movement Disorders Society-European Section (MBS-ES). Part II: Late (complicated) parkinson's disease. *European Journal of Neurology, 13,* 1186–1202.

Huckabee, M. L., & Cannito, M. P. (1999). Outcomes of swallowing rehabilitation in chronic brainstem dysphagia: A retrospective evaluation. *Dysphagia, 14,* 93–109.

Huckabee, M. L., & Pelletier, C. A. (1999). *Management of adult neurogenic dysphagia.* San Diego, CA: Singular.

Huntington Study Group. (1996). Unified Huntington's Disease Rating Scale: Reliability and consistency. *Movement Disorders, 11,* 136–142.

Jankovic, J. (2004). Botulinum toxin in clinical practice. *Journal of Neurology, Neurosurgery and Psychiatry, 75,* 951–957.

Jankovic, J., & Stacy, M. (2007). Medical management of levodopa-associated motor complications in patients with Parkinson's disease. *CNS Drugs, 21,* 677–692.

Jardim, L. B., Pereira, M. L., Silveira, I., Ferro, A., Sequeiros, J., & Giugliani, R. (2001). Neurologic findings in Machado-Joseph disease. *Archives of Neurology, 58,* 899–904.

Jardim, L. B., Silveira, I., Pereira, M. L., Ferro, A., Alonso, I., do Céu Moreira, M., et al. (2001). A survey of spinocerebellar ataxia in South Brazil—66 new cases with Machado-Joseph disease, SCA7, SCA8, or unidentified disease-causing mutations. *Journal of Neurology, 248*, 870-876.

Jones, H. N., Donovan, N. J., Sapienza, C. M., Shrivastav, R., Fernandez, H. H., & Rosenbek, J. C. (2006). Expiratory muscle strength training in the treatment of mixed dysarthria in a patient with Lance-Adams syndrome. *Journal of Medical Speech-Language Pathology, 14*, 207-217.

Josephs, K. A., Ishizawa, T., Tsuboi, Y., Cookson, N., & Dickson, D. W. (2002). A clinicopathological study of vascular progressive supranuclear palsy: A multi-infarct disorder presenting as progressive supranuclear palsy. *Archives of Neurology, 59*, 1597-1601.

Kaat, L. D., Boon, A. J., Kamphorst, W., Ravid, R., Duivenvoorden, H. J., & van Swieten, J. C. (2007). Frontal presentation in progressive supranuclear palsy. *Neurology, 9*, 723-729.

Kagel, M. C., & Leopold, N. A. (1992). Dysphagia in Huntington's disease: A 16-year retrospective. *Dysphagia, 7*, 106-114.

Kahrilas, P. J., Logemann, J. A., & Gibbons, M. S. (1992a). Food intake by maneuver: An extreme compensation for impaired swallowing. *Dysphagia, 7*, 155-159.

Kahrilas, P. J., Logemann, J. A., Krugler, C., & Flanagan, E. (1991). Volitional augmentation of upper esophageal sphincter opening during swallowing. *American Journal of Physiology, 260*, G450-G456.

Kahrilas, P. J., Logemann, J. A., Lin, S., & Ergun, G. A. (1992b). Pharyngeal clearance during swallow: A combined manometric and videofluoroscopic study. *Gastroenterology, 103*, 128-136.

Kahrilas, P. J., Logemann, J. A., Lin, S., Ergun, G. A., & Facchini, R. (1993). Deglutive tongue action: Volume accommodation and bolus propulsion. *Gastroenterology, 104*, 152-162.

Kays, S., & Robbins, J. (2007). Framing oral motor exercise in principles of neural plasticity. *Perspectives on Neurophysiology and Neurogenic Speech and Language Disorders, 17*, 11-17.

Kelly, A. M., Drinnan, M. J., & Leslie, P. (2007). Assessing penetration and aspiration: How do videofluoroscopy and fiberoptic endoscopic evaluation of swallowing compare? *The Laryngoscope, 117*, 1723-1727.

Kelly, A. M., Leslie, P., Beale, T., Payten, C., & Drinnan, M. J. (2006). Fiberoptic endoscopic evaluation of swallowing and videofluoroscopy: Does examination type influence perception of pharyngeal residue severity? *Clinical Otolaryngology, 31*, 425-432.

Kim, J., & Sapienza, C. M. (2005). Implications of expiratory muscle strength training for rehabilitation in the elderly: Tutorial. *Journal of Rehabilitation Research and Development, 42*, 211-224.

Kleim, J. A., & Jones, T. A. (2008). Principles of experience-dependent plasticity: Implication for rehabilitation after brain damage. *Journal of Speech, Language, and Hearing Research, 51*, S227-S239.

Klempir, J., Klempirova, O., Spackova, N., Zidovska, J., & Roth, J. (2006). Unified Huntington's Disease Rating Scale: Clinical practice and a critical approach. *Functional Neurology, 21*, 217-221.

Klockgether, T. (2004). Parkinson's disease: Clinical aspects. *Cell and Tissue Research, 318*, 115-120.

Klockgether, T., Ludtke, R., Kramer, B., Abele, M., Burk, K., Schols, L., et al. (1998). The natural history of degenerative ataxia: A retrospective study of 466 patients. *Brain, 121*, 589-600.

Kompoliti, K., Goetz, C. G., Boeve, B. F., Maraganore, D. M., Ahlskog, J. E., Marsden, C. D., et al. (1998). Clinical presentation and pharmacological therapy in corticobasal degeneration. *Archives of Neurology, 55*, 957-961.

Kondziolka, D., Ong, J. G., Lee, J. Y., Moore, R. Y., Flickinger, J. C., & Lunsford, L. D. (2008). Gamma knife thalamotomy for essential tremor. *Journal of Neurosurgery, 108*, 111-117.

Kosel, M., Sturm, V., Frick, C., Lenartz, D., Zeidler, G., Brodesser, D., et al. (2007). Mood improvement after deep brain stimulation of the internal lobus pallidus for tardive dyskinesia in a patient suffering from major depression. *Journal of Psychiatric Research, 41*, 801-801.

Kozlowski, D. A., James, D. C., & Schallert, T. (1996). Use-dependent exaggeration of neuronal injury following unilateral sensorimotor cortex lesions. *Journal of Neuroscience, 16*, 4776-4786.

Krack, P., Batir, A., Van Blercom, N., Chabardes, S., Fraix, V., Ardoun, C., et al. (2003). Five-year follow-up of bilateral stimulation of the subthalamic nucleus in advanced Parkinson's disease. *New England Journal of Medicine, 349*, 1925-1934.

Kupsch, A., Benecke, R., Muller, J., Trottenberg, T., Schneider, G.-H., Poewe, W., et al. (2006). Pallidal deep-brain stimulation in primary generalized or segmental dystonia. *New England Journal of Medicine, 355*, 1978-1990.

Langmore, S. E. (2003). Evaluation of oropharyngeal dysphagia: Which diagnostic tool is superior? *Current Opinion in Otolaryngology & Head and Neck Surgery, 11*, 485-489.

Langmore, S. E., Schatz, K., & Olson, N. (1988). Fiberoptic endoscopic evaluation of swallowing safety. *Dysphagia, 2*, 216-219.

Langmore, S. E., Terpenning, M. S., Schork, A., Chen, Y., Murray, J. T., Lopatin, D., et al. (1998). Predictors of aspiration pneumonia: How important is dysphagia? *Dysphagia, 13*, 69-81.

Larsen, G. L. (1973). Conservative management for incomplete dysphagia paralytica. *Archives of Physical Medicine and Rehabilitation, 54*, 180-185.

Lazarus, C., Logemann, J. A., & Gibbons, P. (1993). Effects of maneuvers on swallowing function in a dysphagic oral cancer patient. *Head & Neck, 15*, 419-424.

Lazarus, C., Logemann, J. A., Huang, C.-F., & Rademaker, A. W. (2003). Effects of two types of tongue strengthening exercises

in young normals. *Folia Phoniatrica et Logopaedica, 55*, 199-205.

Lazarus, C. L., Logemann, J. A., Pauloski, B. R., Rademaker, A. W., Larson, C. R., Mittal, B. B., et al. (2000). Swallowing and tongue function following treatment for oral and oropharyngeal cancer. *Journal of Speech, Language, and Hearing, 43*, 1011-1023.

Lazarus, C., Logemann, J. A., Song, C. W., Rademaker, A. W., & Kahrilas, P. J. (2002). Effects of voluntary maneuvers on tongue base function for swallowing. *Folia Phoniatrica et Logopaedica, 54*, 171-176.

Leder, S. B., Acton, L. M., Lisitano, H. L., & Murray, J. T. (2005). Fiberoptic endoscopic evaluation of swallowing (FEES) with and without blue-dyed food. *Dysphagia, 20*, 157-162.

Leelamanit, V., Limsakul, C., & Geater, A. (2002). Synchronized electrical stimulation in treating pharyngeal dysphagia. *Laryngoscope, 112*, 2204-2210.

Lefton-Greif, M. A., Crawford, T. O., Winkelstein, J. A., Loughlin, G. M., Zoerner, C. B., Zahurak, M., et al. (2000). Oropharyngeal dysphagia and aspiration in patients with ataxia-telangiectasia. *Journal of Pediatrics, 136*, 225-231.

Leonard, R. J., & Kendall, K. A. (2007). *Dysphagia assessment and treatment planning: A team approach* (2nd ed.). San Diego, CA: Plural.

Leonard, R. J., Kendall, K. A., McKenzie, S., Goncalves, M. I., & Walker, A. (2000). Structural displacements in normal swallowing: A videofluoroscopic study. *Dysphagia, 15*, 146-152.

Leopold, N. A., & Kagel, M. C. (1985). Dysphagia in Huntington's disease. *Archives of Neurology, 42*, 57-60.

Leopold, N. A., & Kagel, M. C. (1997). Dysphagia in progressive supranuclear palsy: Radiologic features. *Dysphagia, 12*, 140-143.

Levine, C. B., Fahrbach, K. R., Siderowf, A. D., Estok, R. P., Ludensky, V. M., & Ross, S. D. (2003). Diagnosis and treatment of Parkinson's disease: A systematic review of the literature. *Evidence Report/Technology Assessment, 57,* 1–4.

Lim, Y. S., & Kennedy, N. J. (2007). Multiple system atrophy as cause of upper airway obstruction. *Anaesthesia, 62,* 1179–1182.

Lim, A., Leow, L., Huckabee, M.-L., Frampton, C., & Anderson, T. (2008). A pilot study of respiration and swallowing integration in Parkinson's disease: "On" and "off" levodopa. *Dysphagia, 23,* 76–81.

Liotti, M.., Ramig, L. O., Vogel, D., New, P., Cook, C. I., Ingham, R. J., et al. (2003). Hypophonia in Parkinson's disease: Neural correlates of voice treatment revealed by PET. *Neurology, 60,* 432–440.

Litvan, I., Agid, Y., Calne, D., Campbell, G., Dubois, B., Duvoisin, R. C., et al. (1996). Clinical research criteria for the diagnosis of progressive supranuclear palsy (Steele-Richardson-Olszewski syndrome): Report of the NINDS-SPSP international workshop. *Neurology, 47,* 1–9.

Litvan, I., Bhatia, K. P., Burn, D. J., Goetz, C. G., Lang, A. E., McKeith, I., et al. (2003). SIC task force appraisal of clinical diagnostic criteria for parkinsonian disorders. *Movement Disorders, 18,* 467–486.

Litvan, I., Sastry, N., & Sonies, B. C. (1997). Characterizing swallowing abnormalities in progressive supranuclear palsy. *Neurology, 48,* 1654–1662.

Lof, G. L., & Robbins, J. (1990). Test-retest variability in normal swallowing. *Dysphagia, 4,* 236-242.

Logemann, J. A. (1983). *Evaluation and treatment of swallowing disorders.* San Diego, CA: College-Hill Press.

Logemann, J. A. (1991). Approaches to management of disordered swallowing. *Bailliere's Clinical Gastroenterology, 5,* 269–280.

Logemann, J. A. (1998). *Evaluation and treatment of swallowing disorders* (2nd ed.). Austin, TX: Pro-Ed.

Logemann, J. A., Gensler, G., Robbins, J., Lindblad, A. S., Brandt, D., Hind, J. A., et al. (2008). A randomized study of three interventions for aspiration of thin liquids in patients with dementia or Parkinson's disease. *Journal of Speech, Language, and Hearing Research, 51,* 173–183.

Logemann, J. A., & Kahrilas, P. J. (1990). Relearning to swallow after stroke—Application of maneuvers and indirect biofeedback: A case study. *Neurology, 40,* 1136–1138.

Logemann, J. A., Kahrilas, P. J., Kobara, M., & Vakil, N. B. (1989). The benefit of head rotation on pharyngoesophageal dysphagia. *Archives of Physical Medicine and Rehabilitation, 70,* 767–771.

Machado, A., Chien, H. F., Deguti, M., Cancado, E., Azevedo, R. S., Scaff, M., et al. (2006). Neurological manifestations in Wilson's disease. Report of 119 cases. *Movement Disorders, 21,* 2192–2196.

Mahapatra, R. K., Edwards, M. J., Schott, J. M., & Bhatia, K. P. (2004). Corticobasal degeneration. *The Lancet Neurology, 3,* 736–743.

Manyam, B. V. (2004). Uncommon forms of tremor. In R. L. Watts & W. C. Koller (Eds.), *Movement disorders: Neurologic principles and practice* (2nd ed., pp. 459–480). New York: McGraw-Hill.

Marin, R. S., Biedrzycki, R. C., & Firinciogullari, S. (1991). Reliability and validity of the apathy evaluation scale. *Psychiatry Review, 38,* 143–162.

Mark, M. H. (2001). Lumping and splitting the Parkinson plus syndromes: Dementia with Lewy bodies, multiple system atrophy, progressive supranuclear palsy, and cortical-basal ganglionic degeneration. *Neurologic Clinics, 19,* 607–627.

Mark, M. H. (2004). Other choreatic disorders. In R. L. Watts & W. C. Koller (Eds.), *Movement disorders: Neurologic principles and practice* (2nd ed., pp. 635–655). New York: McGraw-Hill.

Marrosu, F., Maleci, A., Cocco, E., Puligheddu, M., Barberini, L., & Marrosu, M. G. (2007). Vagal nerve stimulation improves cerebellar tremor and dysphagia in multiple sclerosis. *Multiple Sclerosis, 13,* 1200–1202.

Marshall, F. J. (2004). Clinical features and treatment of Huntington's disease. In R. L. Watts & W. C. Koller (Eds.), *Movement disorders: Neurologic principles and practice*

(2nd ed., pp. 589–601). New York: McGraw-Hill.

Martin-Harris, B., Brodsky, M. B., Michel, Y., Ford, C. L., Walters, B., & Heffner, J. (2005). Breathing and swallowing dynamics across the adult lifespan. *Archives of Otolaryngology–Head & Neck Surgery*, *131*, 762–770.

Martin-Harris, B., Brodsky, M. B., Price, C. C., Michel, Y., Ford, C. L., & Walters, B. (2003). Temporal coordination of pharyngeal and laryngeal dynamics with breathing during swallowing: Single liquid swallows. *Journal of Applied Physiology*, *94*, 1735–1743.

Martin-Harris, B., Michel, Y., & Castell, D. O. (2005). Physiologic model of oropharyngeal swallowing revisited. *Otolaryngology–Head and Neck Surgery*, *133*, 234–240.

Matsumoto, S., Nishimura, M., Shibasaki, H., & Kaji, R. (2003). Epidemiology of primary dystonias in Japan: Comparison with western countries. *Movement Disorders*, *18*, 1196–1198.

McHorney, C. A., Bricker, D. E., Kramer, A. E, Rosenbek, J. C., Robbins, J., Chignell, K. A., et al. (2000). The SWAL-QOL outcomes tool for oropharyngeal dysphagia in adults: I. Conceptual foundation and item development. *Dysphagia*, *15*, 115–121.

McHorney, C. A., Bricker, D. E., Robbins, J., Kramer, A. E., Rosenbek, J. C., & Chignell, K. A. (2000). The SWAL-QOL outcomes tool for oropharyngeal dysphagia in adults: II. Item reduction and preliminary scaling. *Dysphagia*, *15*, 122–133.

McHorney, C. A., Martin-Harris, B., Robbins, J., & Rosenbek, J. (2006). Clinical validity of the SWAL-QOL and SWAL-CARE outcome tools with respect to bolus flow measures. *Dysphagia*, *21*, 141–148.

McHorney, C. A., Robbins, J., Lomax, K., Rosenbek, J. C., Chignell, K. A., Kramer, A. E., et al. (2002). The SWAL-QOL and SWAL-CARE outcomes tool for oropharyngeal dysphagia in adults: III. Documentation of reliability and validity. *Dysphagia*, *17*, 97–114.

Merati, A. L., Heman-Ackah, Y. D., Abaza, M., Altman, K. W., Lulica, L., & Belamowicz, S. (2005). Common movement disorders affecting the larynx: A report from the neurolaryngology committee of the AAO-HNS. *Otolaryngology–Head and Neck Surgery*, *133*, 654–665.

Merlo, I. M., Occhini, A., Pacchetti, C., & Alfonsi, E. (2002). Not paralysis, but dystonia causes stridor in multiple system atrophy. *Neurology*, *58*, 649–652.

Miller, A. J. (1999). *The neuroscientific principles of swallowing and dysphagia*. San Diego, CA: Singular.

Monte, F. S., da Silva-Junior, F. P., Brag-Neto, P., Nobre e Souza, M. A., & de Bruin, V. M. S. (2005). Swallowing abnormalities and dyskinesia in Parkinson's disease. *Movement Disorders*, *4*, 457–462.

Morley, J. E. (2002). Pathophysiology of anorexia. *Clinics in Geriatric Medicine*, *18*, 661–673.

Mosier, K., & Bereznaya, I. (2001). Parallel cortical networks for volitional control of swallowing in humans. *Experimental Brain Research*, *140*, 280–289.

Muller, J., Wenning, G. K., Verny, M., McKee, A., Chaudhuri, K. R., Jellinger, K., et al. (2001). Progression of dysarthria and dysphagia in postmortem-confirmed parkinsonian disorders. *Archives of Neurology*, *58*, 259–264.

Murray, J., & Musson, N. (2005). Understanding dysphagia (Version 1.0) [CD-ROM]. Gainesville, FL: North Florida Foundation for Research and Education, Inc.

Nagaya, M., Kachi, T., Yamada, T., & Sumi, Y. (2004). Videofluorographic observations on swallowing in patients with dysphagia due to neurodegenerative diseases. *Nagoya Journal of Medical Science*, *67*, 17–23.

Nath, U., Ben-Shlomo, Y., Thomson, R. G., Lees, A. J., & Burn, D. J. (2003). Clinical features and natural history of progressive supranuclear palsy: A clinical cohort study. *Neurology*, *60*, 910–916.

The National Dysphagia Diet Task Force. (2002). *The National Dysphagia Diet: Standardization of clinical care*. Chicago: American Dietetic Association.

Neumann, S., Reich, S., Buchholz, D., Purcell, L., & Jones, B. (1996). Progressive supranuclear palsy (PSP): Characteristics of dysphagia in 14 patients [Abstract]. *Dysphagia, 11*, 164.

Nilsson, H., Ekberg, O., Olsson, R., & Hindfelt, B. (1996). Swallowing in hereditary sensory ataxia. *Dysphagia, 11*, 140-143.

Nussbaum, R. L., & Ellis, C. E. (2003). Alzheimer's disease and Parkinson's disease. *New England Journal of Medicine, 348*, 1356-1364.

Nutt, J. G., Muenter, M. D., Aronson, A., Kurland, L. T., & Melton, L. J. (1988). Epidemiology of focal and generalized dystonia in Rochester, Minnesota. *Movement Disorders, 3*, 188-194.

Oder, W., Grimm, G., Kollegger, H., Ferenci, P., Schneider, B., & Deecke, L. (1991). Neurological and neuropsychiatric spectrum of Wilson's disease: A prospective study of 45 cases. *Journal of Neurology, 238*, 281-287.

Oertel, W. H., & Moller, J. C. (2004). Rare degenerative syndromes associated with parkinsonism. In R. L. Watts & W. C. Koller (Eds.), *Movement disorders: Neurologic principles and practice* (2nd ed., pp. 403-420). New York: McGraw-Hill.

Ohame, Y., Ogura, M., Kitahara, S., Karaho, T., & Inouye, T. (1998). Effects of head rotation on pharyngeal function during normal swallow. *Annals of Otology, Rhinology, and Laryngology, 107*, 344-348.

Ostergaard, K., Sunde, N., & Dupont, E. (2002). Effects of bilateral stimulation of the subthalamic nucleus in patients with severe Parkinson's disease and motor fluctuations. *Movement Disorders, 17*, 693-700.

Papapetropoulos, S., & Singer, C. (2006). Eating dysfunction associated with oromandibular dystonia: Clinical characteristics and treatment considerations. *Head & Face Medicine, 2*, 47.

Paslawski, T., Duffy, J. R., & Vernino, S. (2005). Speech and language findings associated with paraneoplastic cerebellar degeneration. *American Journal of Speech-Language Pathology, 14*, 200-207.

Paulson, H., & Ammache, Z. (2001). Ataxia and hereditary disorders. *Movement Disorders, 19*, 759-782.

Pekmezovic, T., Ivanovic, N., Svetel, M., Nalic, D., Smiljkovic, T., Raicevic, R., et al. (2003). Prevalence of primary late-onset focal dystonia in the Belgrade population. *Movement Disorders, 18*, 1389-1392.

Perlman, A., & Van Deale, D. (1993). Simultaneous videoendoscopic and ultrasound measures of swallowing. *Journal of Medical Speech-Language Pathology, 1*, 223-232.

Pfeiffer, R. F. (2004). Wilson's disease. In R. L. Watts & W. C. Koller (Eds.), *Movement disorders: Neurologic principles and practice* (2nd ed., pp. 779-797). New York: McGraw-Hill.

Pouderoux, P., & Kahrilas, P. J. (1995). Deglutitive tongue force modulation by volition, volume, and viscosity in humans. *Gastroenterology, 108*, 1418-1426.

Power, M., Fraser, C., Hobson, A., Rothwell, J. C., Mistry, S., Nicholson, D. A., et al. (2004). Changes in pharyngeal corticobulbar excitability and swallowing behavior after oral stimulation. *American Journal of Physiology-Gastrointestinal and Liver Physiology, 286*, G45-G50.

Power, M. L., Fraser, C. H., Hobson, A., Singh, S., Tyrell, P., Nicholson, D. A., et al. (2006). Evaluating oral stimulation as a treatment for dysphagia after stroke. *Dysphagia, 21*, 49-55.

Powers, S. K., & Howley, E. T. (2003). Exercise physiology: Theory and application to fitness and performance (5th ed.). Boston: McGraw-Hill.

Ramio-Torrenta, L., Gomez, E., & Genis, D. (2006). Swallowing in degenerative ataxias. *Journal of Neurology, 253*, 875-881.

Rasley, A., Logemann, J. A., Kahrilas, P. J., Rademaker, A. W., Pauloski, B. R., & Dodds, W. J. (1993). Prevention of barium aspiration during videofluoroscopic swallowing studies: Value of change in posture. *American Journal of Roentgenology, 160*, 1005-1009.

Risch, N., de Leon, D., Ozelius, L., Kramer, P., Almasy, L., Singer, B., et al. (1995). Genetic analysis of idiopathic torsion dystonia in Ashkenazi Jews and their recent descent from a small founder population. *Nature Genetics, 11*, 13-15.

Riski, J. E., Horner, J., & Nashold, B. S. (1990). Swallowing function in patients with spasmodic torticollis. *Neurology, 40*, 1443-1445.

Robbins, J., Gangnon, R. E., Theis, S. M., Kays, S. A., Hewitt, A. L., & Hind, J. A. (2005). The effects of lingual exercise on swallowing in older adults. *Journal of the American Geriatric Society, 53*, 1483-1489.

Robbins, J., Kays, S. A., Gangmon, R. E., Hind, J. A., Hewitt, A. L., Gentry, L. R., et al. (2007). The effects of lingual exercise in stroke patients with dysphagia. *Archives of Physical Medicine and Rehabilitation, 88*, 150-158.

Robbins, J., & Levine, R. L. (1993). Swallowing after lateral medullary syndrome plus. *Clinics in Communication Disorders, 3*, 45-55.

Robbins, J., Levine, R., Wood, J., Roecker, E., & Luschei, E. (1995). Age effects on lingual pressure generation as a risk factor for dysphagia. *The Journals of Gerontology. Series A, Biological Sciences and Medical Sciences, 50*, M257-M262.

Robin, D. A., Goel, A., Somodi, L. B., & Luschei, E. S. (1992). Tongue strength and endurance: Relation to highly skilled movements. *Journal of Speech and Hearing Research, 35*, 1239-1245.

Robin, D. A., Somodi, L. B., & Luschei, E. S. (1991). Measurement of tongue strength and endurance in normal and articulation disordered adults. In C. A. Moore, K. M. Yorkston, & D. R. Buekelman (Eds.), *Dysarthria and apraxia of speech: Perspectives on management* (pp. 173-184). Baltimore: Paul H. Brookes.

Ropper, A. H., & Brown, R. H. (2005). *Adams and Victor's principles of neurology* (8th ed.). New York: McGraw-Hill.

Rosenbek, J. C., & Jones, H. N. (2006). Dysphagia in patients with motor speech disorders. In G. Weismer (Ed.), *Motor speech disorders* (pp 221-259). San Diego, CA: Plural.

Rosenbek, J. C., Robbins, J., Fishback, B., & Levine, R. L. (1991). Effects of thermal application on dysphagia after stroke. *Journal of Speech and Hearing Research, 34*, 1257-1268.

Rosenbek, J. C., Robbins, J. A., Roecker, E. B., Coyle, J. L., & Wood, J. L. (1996). A penetration-aspiration scale. *Dysphagia, 11*, 93-98.

Rosenbek, J. C., Robbins, J., Willford, W. O., Kirk, G., Schlitz, A., Sowell, T. W., et al. (1998). Comparing treatment intensities of tactile-thermal application. *Dysphagia, 13*, 1-9.

Rosenbek, J. C., Roecker, E. B., Wood, J. L., & Robbins, J. (1996). Thermal application reduces the duration of stage transition in dysphagia after stroke. *Dysphagia, 11*, 225-233.

Rub, U., Brunt, R., Del Turco, D., de Vost, R. A. I., Gierga, K., Paulson, H., et al. (2003). Guidelines for the pathoanatomical examination of the lower brain stem in ingestive and swallowing disorders and its application to a dysphagic spinocerebellar ataxia type 3 patient. *Neuropathology and Applied Neurobiology, 29*, 1-13.

Saleem, A. F., Sapienza, C. M, & Okun, M. S. (2005). Respiratory muscle strength training: Treatment and response duration in a patient with early idiopathic Parkinson's disease. *NeuroRehabilitation, 20*, 323-333.

Santens, P., Vonck, K., De Letter, M., Van Driessche, K., Sieben, A., De Reuck, J., et al. (2006). Deep brain stimulation of the internal pallidum in multiple system atrophy. *Parkinsonism and Related Disorders, 12*, 181-183.

Sapienza, C. M., Davenport, P. W., & Martin, A. D. (2002). Expiratory muscle training improves pressure support in high school band students. *Journal of Voice, 16*, 495-501.

Sasco, A. J., Paffenbarger, R. S., Gendre, I., & Wing, A. L. (1992). The role of physical exercise in the occurrence of Parkinson's disease. *Archives of Neurology, 49*, 360-365.

Schneider, S. A., Aggarwal, A., Bhatt, M., Dupont, E., Tisch, S., Limousin, P., et al. (2006). Severe tongue protrusion dystonia: Clinical syndromes and possible treatment. *Neurology, 67,* 940–943.

Shaker, R., Easterling, C., Kern, M., Nitschke, T., Massey, B., Daniels, S., et al. (2002). Rehabilitation of swallowing by exercise in tube-fed patients with pharyngeal dysphagia secondary to abnormal UES opening. *Gastroenterology, 122,* 1314–1321.

Shaker, R., Kern, M., Bardan, E., Taylor, A., Stewart, E., Hoffmann, R., et al. (1997). Augmentation of deglutitive upper esophageal sphincter opening in the elderly by exercise. *American Journal of Physiology, 272,* G1518–1522.

Shaw, G., Sechtem, P., Searl, J., Keller, K., Taib, A., & Dowdy, E. (2007). Transcutaneous neuromuscular electrical stimulation (VitalStim) curative therapy for severe dysphagia: Myth or reality? *Annals of Otology, Rhinology, and Laryngology, 116,* 36–44.

Shulman, L. M., Minagar, A., & Weiner, W. J. (2004). Multiple-system atrophy. In R. L. Watts & W. C. Koller (Eds.), *Movement disorders: Neurologic principles and practice* (2nd ed., pp. 359–369). New York: McGraw-Hill.

Silverman, E. P., Sapienza, C. M., Saleem, A., Carmichael, C., Davenport, P. W., Hoffman-Ruddy, B., et al. (2006). Tutorial on maximum inspiratory and expiratory mouth pressures in individuals with idiopathic Parkinson disease (IPD) and the preliminary results of an expiratory muscle strength training program. *NeuroRehabilitation, 21,* 71–79.

Sjostrom, A.-C., Holmberg, B., & Strang, P. (2002). Parkinson-plus patients—An unknown group with severe symptoms. *Journal of Neuroscience Nursing, 34,* 314–319.

Smith, A. D., & Zigmond, M. J. (2003). Can the brain be protected through exercise? Lessons from an animal model of parkinsonism. *Experimental Neurology, 184,* 31–39.

Solomon, N. P., Robin, D. A., Lorell, D. M., Rodnitzky, R. L., & Luschei, E. S. (1994). Tongue function testing in Parkinson's disease. In J. A. Till, K. M. Yorkston, & D. R. Beukelman (Eds.), *Motor Speech Disorders* (pp. 147–160). Baltimore: Paul H. Brookes.

Solomon, N. P., Robin, D. A., & Luschei, E. S. (2000). Strength, endurance, and stability of the tongue and hand in Parkinson's disease. *Journal of Speech, Language, and Hearing research, 43,* 256–267.

Sonies, B. (1992). Swallowing and speech disturbances. In I. Litvan & Y. Agid (Eds.), *Progressive supranuclear palsy: Clinical and research approaches* (pp. 240–253). New York: Oxford University Press,

Stacy, M. (2000). Pharmacotherapy for advanced Parkinson's disease. *Pharmacotherapy, 20,* 8S–16S.

Stacy, M. A. (2007). Botulinum toxin in the treatment of dystonia. In M. A. Stacy (Ed.), *Handbook of dystonia* (pp. 355–370). New York: Informa Healthcare USA.

Stein, R. B., Chong, S. L., James, K. B., Kido, A., Bell, G. J., Tubman, L. A., et al. (2002). Electrical stimulation for therapy and mobility after spinal cord injury. *Progress in Brain Research, 137,* 27–34.

Stover, N. P., Wainer, B. H., & Watts, R. L. (2004). Corticobasal degeneration. In R. L. Watts & W. C. Koller (Eds.), *Movement disorders: Neurologic principles and practice* (2nd ed., pp. 763–778). New York: McGraw-Hill.

Sun, B., Chen, S., Zhan, S., Le, W., & Krahl, S. E. (2007). Subthalamic nucleus stimulation for primary dystonia and tardive dystonia. *Acta Neurochirurgica, 97,* 207–214.

Suzuki, M., Asada, Y., Ito, J., Hayashi, K., Inoue, H., & Kitano, H. (2003). Activation of cerebellum and basal ganglia on volitional swallowing detected by functional magnetic resonance imaging. *Dysphagia, 18,* 71–77.

Tagliati, M., Shils, J. C. S., & Alterman, R. (2004). Deep brain stimulation for dystonia. *Expert Review of Medical Devices, 1,* 33–41.

Tarsy, D. (2000). Tardive dyskinesia. *Current Treatment Options in Neurology*, *2*, 205–214.

Tarsy, D., Apetauerova, D., Ryan, P., & Norregaard, T. (2003). Adverse effects of subthalamic nucleus DBS in a patient with multiple system atrophy. *Neurology*, *61*, 247–249.

Thobois, S., Broussolle, E., Toureill, L., & Vial, C. (2001). Severe dysphagia after botulinum toxin injection for cervical dystonia in multiple system atrophy. *Movement Disorders*, *16*, 764–765.

Toda, H., Hamani, C., & Lozano, A. (2004). Deep brain stimulation in the treatment of dyskinesia and dystonia. *Neurosurgical Focus*, *17*, 9–13.

Trejo, A., Boll, M.-C., Alonso, E., Ochoa, A., & Velasquez, L. (2005). Use of oral nutritional supplements in patients with Huntington's disease. *Nutrition*, *21*, 889–894.

Troche, M. S., Sapienza, C. M., & Rosenbek, J. C. (2008). Effects of bolus consistency of timing and safety of swallow in patients with Parkinson's disease. *Dysphagia*, *23*, 26–32.

Tuite, P. J., & Lang, A. E. (1996). Severe and prolonged dysphagia complicating botulinum toxin A injections for dystonia in Machado-Joseph disease. *Neurology*, *46*, 846.

Vanacore, N., Bonifati, V., Colosimo, C., Fabbrini, G., De Michele, G., Marconi, R., et al. (2001). Epidemiology of multiple system atrophy. SEGAP Consortium. European Study Group on Atypical Parkinsonisms. *Neurological Sciences*, *22*, 101–103.

Veis, S., Logemann, J. A., & Colangelo, L. (2000). Effects of three techniques on maximum posterior movement of the tongue base. *Dysphagia*, *15*, 142–145.

Victor, M., & Ropper, A. H. (2001). *Principles of neurology* (7th ed.). New York: McGraw-Hill.

Vidailhet, M., Vercueil, L., Houeto, J.-L., Krystkowiak, P., Benabid, A.-L., Cornu, P., et al. (2005). Bilateral deep-brain stimulation of the globus pallidus in primary generalized dystonia. *New England Journal of Medicine*, *352*, 459–467.

Volkman, J., Sturm, V., Weiss, P., Kappler, J., Voges, J., Koulousakis, et al. (1998). Bilateral high-frequency stimulation if the internal globus pallidus in advanced Parkinson's disease. *Annals of Neurology*, *44*, 953–961.

Wang, X.-H., Cheng, F., Zhang, F., Li, X. C., Kong, L. B., Li, G. Q., et al. (2005). Living-related liver transplantation for Wilson's disease. *Transplants International*, *18*, 651–656.

Watanabe, H., Saito, Y., Terao, S., Ando, T., Kachi, T., Mukai, E., et al. (2002). Progression and prognosis in multiple system atrophy: An analysis of 230 Japanese patients. *Brain*, *125*, 1070–1083.

Welch, M. V., Logemann, J. A., Rademaker, A. W., & Kahrilas, P. J. (1993). Changes in pharyngeal dimensions effected by chin tuck. *Archives of Physical Medicine and Rehabilitation*, *74*, 178–181.

Wenning, G. K., Litvan, I., Jankovic, J., Granata, R., Nangone, C. A., McKee, A., et al. (1998). Natural history and survival of 14 patients with corticobasal degeneration confirmed at postmortem examination. *Journal of Neurology, Neurosurgery and Psychiatry*, *64*, 184–189.

Wenning, G. K., & Quinn, N. P. (1997). Parkinsonism. Multiple system atrophy. *Balliere's Clinical Neurology*, *6*, 187–204.

Wheeler, K. M., Chiara, T., & Sapienza, C. M. (2007). Surface electromyographic activity of the submental muscles during swallow and expiratory pressure threshold tasks. *Dysphagia*, *22*, 108–116.

Wilkins, R. H., & Brody, I. A. (1971). Neurological Classics XXXVI. Wilson's disease (S. A. Wilson). *Archives of Neurology*, *25*, 179–185.

Wilmot, G. R., & Subramony, S. H. (2004). The molecular genetics of the ataxia. In R. L. Watts & W. C. Koller (Eds.), *Movement disorders: Neurologic principles and practices* (2nd ed., pp. 705–722). New York: McGraw-Hill.

Yorkston, K. M., Miller, R. M., & Strand, E. A. (2004). *Management of speech and swallowing in degenerative diseases* (2nd ed.).

San Antonio, TX: Communication Skill Builders.

Zachary, V., & Mills, R. H. (2000). Nutritional evaluation and laboratory values in dysphagia management. In R. H. Mills (Ed.), *Evaluation of dysphagia in adults: Expanding the diagnostic options* (pp. 179–206). Austin, TX: Pro-ED.

Zesiewicz, T. A., Elble, R., Louis, E. D., Hauser, R. A., Sullivan, K. L, Dewey, R. B., et al. (2005). Practice parameter: Therapies for essential tremor. Report of the Quality Standards Subcommittee of the American Academy of Neurology. *Neurology, 64*, 2008–2020.

Zilber, N., Korczyn, A. D., Kahana, E., Fried, K., & Alter, M. (1984). Inheritance of idiopathic torsion dystonia among Jews. *Journal of Medical Genetics, 21*, 13–20.

Index

Note: page numbers in **bold type** reference non-text information.